Surviving Cancer

A Story of Hope

By T. E. Bradford

Dedication

To all those out there who are reading this book because they or someone they love are dealing with cancer, I hope that the words provide insight, understanding, compassion, strength and hope.

This book is for you.

Intro

Hi. My name is Tracy. I have cancer.

Saying it out loud kind of sucks. Hopefully at some point soon I can say I *had* cancer. Why, you might ask, am I writing this book? Well, I'm a writer. It's what I do. Plus, it's therapy for me. I wrote all through my growing up years, and I feel as if this helped make me a better balanced kid. I had an outlet. In hindsight, I realize that this is a blessing from God. He gave me something that feels like a little piece of magic. I can fall into my stories and escape for a while. I can write about things that bother me, and then they don't hurt so badly. I can write about things I love, and leave a legacy. It's a pretty amazing thing.

So yes, I'm writing about cancer. I want to write an open, honest account of what it feels like, what I go through, what family and friends go through... all of it. Something tells me I'm supposed to do this. I need to do this.

Cancer can be a very hopeless thing. I belong to a support group, and I see story after story of people without hope; people who have lost family, love, body parts, security, dexterity, energy, humanity... themselves. Cancer has taken all this from them. I am one of the lucky ones. I have hope. I have that because I know that even if I lose this battle, I can still cling to God's promises. He already conquered death. How anyone could face something like this without faith is beyond me.

So by writing, I hope to share my journey, share my story, and most importantly share my hope with others.

Here goes nothing.

Life Changer

A year ago my doctor told me I was anemic. I wasn't really too concerned about that. I'd been anemic before. There were lots of possible reasons for it. I had been raised not eating much meat. We weren't strictly vegetarian, but I definitely didn't eat as much meat as most people, especially red meat. I don't eat many green vegetables either. Terrible I know, but true. Also, I have always had fairly heavy menses. That got worse as I got older, so it wasn't a stretch to say I was anemic. Still, my doctor wanted me to have a colonoscopy.

Feeling more than a little rebellious, I saw the GI (*Gastroenterologist or Gastro Intestinal*) doc. He agreed with me. He was surprised my doctor wanted me to have a colonoscopy. I explained all of the possible reasons for my anemia, and noted that I was considering a uterine ablation procedure to help fix the heavy menses. My OBGYN had already said that he thought the anemia could very likely be from that. GI doc agreed.

So there. In your face, Doc.

I asked the GI what would happen if this was something else. Would waiting to see if the ablation fixed the anemia be a danger? GI doc said no. It takes ten years for colon polyps to turn into cancer, so having the ablation and waiting to see would not do much of anything.

Happy dance!

No colonoscopy for this chick. Not if I could help it.

I did just what I wanted. I did the ablation. I blew off the GI stuff. I told my doctor two out of three doctors agreed with me, not her. Not in so many words of course, but that was the gist of it.

The ablation went really well. All signs of menses went away. I haven't had to deal with one since. Bleeding gone. I was loving it. Right up until my doctor told me I was still anemic. What? When did we even do blood work? That was crazy. How long did it take to for the blood cells to regenerate? I reiterated all my original arguments.

My doctor said, and I quote, "We have to assume colon cancer until proven otherwise."

Wow.

That was a very bad day. I went home and tore the heads off my family for no reason. Then I hid in my garage and cried for a while. When I finally told my husband why I was so upset, what the doctor had said, he was angry. Even if she was concerned she shouldn't have put it like that. I admitted I was still anemic, and that scared me. What if she was right? I had to have a colonoscopy, just to be safe. And right after we found out it was nothing I was going to fire my doctor.

The GI set up my colonoscopy, but with no history of colon cancer in my family he was fairly confident this was nothing worse than hemorrhoids.

March 4, 2016 I had my colonoscopy. I woke up from the anesthesia just as they were finishing, and heard the GI doctor say, "now I wish I'd made her do this a year ago."

Oh crap. Was he talking about me? God, I hope he wasn't talking about me. Maybe he was discussing another patient. Someone else. Not me. Right?

Then I was waking up in recovery, and my husband was there, and GI doctor was there looking very serious. He did find something, he explained, and he did think it was cancer.

Long pause here, because I think the world stopped for a moment. Or it flipped inside-out. Or something.

I think I asked some questions. Maybe I nodded my head, or said mm-hmm a few times. Something like that. I was fairly composed. GI doctor showed us pictures of the mass. My mass. He gave me a print out of the pictures. The mass was ten centimeters. How big is that? About four inches, apparently. The width of my fist across the knuckles. I had a four inch mass inside me. GI doctor said he would be recommending me to a surgeon and an oncologist. He was so sorry.

We left in a daze.

Sometime later, my hubby admitted to me he'd planned to take me out to lunch to celebrate. Instead, we drove home mostly silent and probably in shock. Neither of us was hungry now.

Then it hit me.

My doctor had been right. Blast it all. Right then, right at that moment, I hated her for it. I hated that she'd been right, and I was wrong. I hated she'd made me face the possibility and then the reality of it. Maybe I'd just never go back to her. How could I face that? How could I not just eat crow, but have cancer too? Man. This sucked.

The calls started coming in pretty quickly. Lots of appointments were set up: One with a surgeon because the mass had to come out; another with an oncologist because I might need chemotherapy.

Holy crap.

This is the moment where the reality of your own mortality really slaps you upside the head. It's one thing to imagine it. To think about it in passing, rhetorically, when you can still believe it's far away. It's another to know that you literally may not be around a year or two from now. That you might stop living, and breathing and being. But honestly, the scary stuff isn't about yourself, it's about your family. My son was not even in Kindergarten yet. My husband relied on me for our primary income and our health insurance. We never saved up enough to be financially prepared for something like this. Leaving them behind might mean losing the house and any sense of security they might have.

That was the hard part. I am a Mom. It's who I am more than any other role in my life. Taking care of my family is what makes me... *me*. The idea of not being able to do that was enormous. It was brutal.

I looked up some things online, but there was a lot of scary information out there.

The hardest part was reading stories about cancer patients who were also moms and dads of small kids. One story was about a girl who died of colon cancer really young, and whose family started a foundation in her honor.

Wait... that was supposed to be uplifting?

The story talked about her young children asking their Grandpa if he thought Mommy was out of pain now up in Heaven, and that they missed her.

Ripped. My. Heart. Out.

This hit too close to home. Quick, close that page.

Then I chanced on something that turned out to be one of the best things I could have discovered. I found a colon cancer support group. New people are greeted with "Sorry you have to be here, but glad you found us!" – and ain't that the truth. None of them wanted to be here, but finding them changed everything.

I read some posts and some of them were a little scary but mostly they were informative and inspiring. I needed to know more. One thing I figured out quick was that I didn't want this to be Stage IV. That was *super* scary territory. I joined the group and started posting immediately. Here's an excerpt from my first post, with info from my colonoscopy results:

"Colonoscopy yesterday (3/4/16) reveals 1 - 1cm Polyp in the descending colon, which was removed, and 1 - 10cm Mass in the sigmoid colon to distal descending colon, which was injected and biopsied, believed to be cancer.

After reading some of the posts on size, I see that it can be bigger and lower stage, smaller and further stage, etc., but I still feel pretty daunted by having a mass so large. Some of my questions are: does this diagnosis mean it's definitely cancer, or do I have to wait for the biopsy results? Also, am I right to assume that with a 10cm mass, the lowest I can hope for is Stage II, or is it at least Stage III automatically?

I know you've all probably heard this a thousand times already, so thank you ahead of time for being so gracious to a new nervous Nelly (or Tracy in my case)."

Age 46

Mom of a soon-to-be 5-yr-old boy

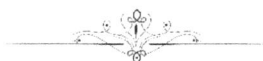

The responses to my post began pouring in. Here was a group of people who had gone through much the same thing I was going through, and they had advice. They had information. They quickly explained that with colon cancer, size has *nothing* whatsoever to do with staging. You could have a HUGE mass and be Stage I. You could have a tiny mass and be Stage IV. They kindly and compassionately told me not to surf the net, not to believe half of what I read because it was either outdated or flat out wrong, and to try to breathe and sit tight until we could learn more.

They were compassionate. They were helpful. They used terms I needed a dictionary to understand (which they thankfully had a whole topic dedicated to so that people can look up terms and acronyms).

For the first time, I started to pull back from the brink of panic. I was still freaking out, but I was getting some of my control back, trickle by trickle.

Okay, breathe Tracy.

One of the members told me, "You're not going to die today, or tomorrow, or the next day, so just try to take a deep breath."

After a few days, still feeling really good and healthy (which was kind of weird considering I had this thing inside me), I did start to feel a bit of normalcy creeping back in. I bulked up on information because it made me feel more stable. It gave me some of my power back in a situation that felt mostly powerless.

I shared with the support group that being a Mom was the hardest part, not knowing what this was going to do to my son. In private, I cried because I had always planned to be there as he grew up. I wanted to teach him about God, and having faith. Who was going to teach him that if I wasn't around to do it?

Then one of the folks on the support group sent me a response that literally changed my perspective one hundred and eighty degrees. She said that she was a mom of two young children also, and while this experience was maybe making them grow up a little quicker than she would have liked, they actually enjoyed having "mom duty" and getting to take care of her. She was using this, she told me, as an opportunity to show them what it meant to take care of family.

And just like that, it clicked.

This was my opportunity to show my son first-hand what it meant to rely on God. I could show him rather than tell him what faith was. Why I had hope. This was my chance to be a living example for my child.

There's a song by Babbie Mason and Rodney Griffin that says, "Turn every test into a testimony" and that is exactly what I decided to do.

Preparing for Battle

I'm not usually one to share the things that are more private in my life. I tend to shy away from that.

Cancer was different.

Right from the get-go I didn't hold back. I couldn't. I knew that this was a battle I was going to face, and I had to pull my resources and get ready to fight. As soon as I found out I called my boss, since there would be a lot of new appointments coming up fast.

He said (and I quote), "First priority is *you*, second priority is *you*, and nothing else matters."

Honestly, when he said that, it was the first time since actual diagnosis that I cried. I realized I was truly blessed. After working for over seven years at an organization where I felt as though my very best wasn't nearly good enough, where after several years of glowing reviews and quick advancements I was suddenly told I wasn't cutting it, the opportunity for my current job opened up. I could almost feel the doors just flying open. Everything fell into place without me even having believed I would really consider it. I felt led to take the job I'm in now. So I accepted it. And right after I gave my notice at my old job, wondering if I was crazy and doing something insane, I turned on the radio. I listen to the gospel music channel on satellite radio. It's like a lifeline for me. As soon as I turned it on that day, I caught the end of a conversation and these words: "Sometimes God opens a door and we just have to walk through it."

So yes, I know I'm blessed to have this job, and this boss. The support here has been incredible. In the time I've worked here, I've made more friends than I did in the seven plus years at my previous job. Here, I have people who hug me, ask about me, even pray for me.

Not everyone facing cancer is nearly so lucky. I've read story after story about people who lost their jobs, got crap from their jobs or just couldn't deal with the way people were treating them. Insurance nightmares, jobs mysteriously downsized, it's a crappy but stark reality. Did God place me in this job knowing full well what I needed and to make sure I had it?

You bet He did!

I believe that with all my heart.

After letting work know what would be coming, I called my family members and let them know. Then I posted the info online. I didn't want there to be any surprises. I would have to focus on getting myself better for a while, and I wanted to be sure everyone knew.

Just like with the support group, supportive prayer-filled responses flowed in. I heard from people I hadn't talked to in years, some whose kindness and friendship I probably didn't deserve, but they chose to respond anyway. People that I had no idea were fellow believers were ready to lift me up in prayer. My name was added to prayer list after prayer list. If you've ever felt this kind of outpouring, then you know how absolutely humbling and amazing it can be. If not, I hope that someday you have the chance to experience it.

I asked for everyone to pray that the results of my CT scan came back clear. That was the next step on this journey. Scan, then an exam by the surgeon to ensure we were ready for surgery. The CT scan would show whether or not the cancer had metastasized to any other organs (called "distant mets"). Colon cancer has a propensity to spread to liver and lungs, so those were the areas of focus, although they look at your whole chest and abdomen. If my cancer had spread to any of these other areas, I would be an immediate Stage IV.

The anxiety began to build.

My results were scheduled to come in on or before the appointment with my surgeon. This exam, a sigmoidoscopy, would confirm the location of the mass from my original colonoscopy.

The day of the exam came. When they prepped me, my blood pressure was 199/119. I was trying to stay calm, but my body knew better. The nurse that came to ask all the prep questions went through the list. Any heart problems? Been to a foreign country recently? Any metal parts installed in my body? It almost made me feel pretty healthy being able to say no to all of these things. Then she asks, "Any history of cancer?"

"Well, not until now," I answered, not exactly sure whether I could call it a 'history' yet.

Man, you should have seen her face. She had apparently either not been privy to my chart, or hadn't paid attention to it.

"Oh, I'm sorry," she fumbled. "You know, if you're going to be getting chemo, they can install a port!" She was happy to share with me.

Oookaaay...

Add another few numbers to my blood pressure, thank you very much.

They wheeled me in for the procedure, and there was my surgeon. Seeing her was very reassuring.

I haven't mentioned it yet, but on meeting this woman both my husband and I had gained an immediate appreciation for her. She not only took the time to speak with us, she showed us pictures of where things were located in the body, where my tumor was, how the surgery would work, what to expect, etc. She let us ask questions. She took her time. Then she very confidently told us she was really good at what she did. It was all she did, she did a lot of them, and she was good at it. Her kindness as well as obvious competence was very reassuring.

In spite of being the deliverer of bad news, I also liked my GI doctor. From the first time I met him I had sense of confidence in him that I still have today. The fact that he recommended my surgeon, who was obviously an all-star made me trust both of them that much more with my care.

When dealing with cancer, you end up with a whole team of doctors. The better they can work together, the better for you! One thing my support group stressed over and over again was to make sure your surgeon is Board Certified as a Colo-Rectal Surgeon, not just a general surgeon. This is important because only surgeons who specialize in this particular type of surgery, who do it day in and day out, can make quick decision on the fly during surgery that might impact you long-term. You don't want to put that kind of thing in the hands of someone who does various types of surgery, and may have only done a handful of the type specific to colo-rectal. This is particularly important if it's rectal cancer, and you might need an ileostomy. So if anyone is reading this and is in this situation, please check to be sure. It's important!

Most of the folks in the support group also encourage getting a second opinion, especially if you're at all unclear of why a certain method will be used, or whether you should be having surgery before or after other types of treatment, etc.

The bottom line is, you have to make sure you trust and like your doctors, that you have full confidence in them. You're going to be working with them a LOT, and you have to trust them with your life. I already trusted my GI, and now I trusted my surgeon as well. I was extremely fortunate.

As they got ready to put me under for my sigmoidoscopy, I asked my surgeon if we'd be getting the results of the CT scan.

"Yes, we have them already," she said to me, "they're all good!"

That was the last thing I heard before anesthesia took over.

Blood pressure before procedure: 199/119.

Blood pressure after procedure: 140/80.

Yeah, it was big. This was the first bit of good news we'd gotten since the initial diagnosis. The pathology from the biopsy had come back positive for Invasive Adenocarcinoma. We'd chosen not to share that tidbit with friends and family until after the results of the CT scan. We figured that telling them that first would only make them worry, and getting the results of the CT scan would provide a clearer idea of what we were dealing with. Of course, it also allowed us to give some good news along with the bad. This is how the cancer process seems to work. You get some good news, you get some bad news. There are lots of ups and downs. Mostly downs, you might think, but it's surprising what ends up being good news once you've faced something like cancer.

So now we were able to take another deep breath. It was like living in really fast or really slow motion. One breath here, another breath there. In between we held it.

The surgeon gave us a few bits of additional info that day. One was that while the CT scan was clear, it did show something might be going on with my bladder. I'd need to see an urologist for that before surgery so that we could know whether anything additional should be incorporated into the procedure. In other words, I might have bladder stones. As I found out later, the scan results noted "debris" in my bladder. As a lifelong storm enthusiast, I almost found that kind of cool. I had my very own debris. Also, my liver appeared slightly enlarged. Easily explained by irritation from the tumor, or possibly because I was overweight. Duly noted.

They look for all of this prior to surgery because they only want to have to open you up and have you under anesthesia once if they can help it. Taking care of any / all other circumstances at once is optimum. Fortunately, a visit to the urologist confirmed that my debris was just that. Debris.

"If a snowball is bladder stones," my urologist explained, "then what you have is snow."

Nothing to worry about, nothing to need additional surgery for. Hooray!

During the sigmoidoscopy the surgeon also found that the mass was not in the central sigmoid, but actually closer to the descending. This was a good thing, as it meant the mass was farther away from the rectum, meaning I didn't have to worry about an ileostomy (poop bag, as we CRC veterans call it). Also, the mass was slightly smaller than originally noted at nine centimeters vs. ten.

So, there it was. Next stop would be surgery, and then we'd find out for sure what was going on.

Oh, but first there was the wee matter of a visit to the Oncologist.

Oscar

As you might imagine, no part about going to an oncologist is fun. Just the word is kind of intimidating, let alone the building or medical center.

Still, this was just an initial consultation. Another deep breath.

I walked in, and the first thing I saw was a huge reception area. Lots of people have cancer. It's a booming business. The next thing I noticed was the huge in-house pharmacy on the right, and the little shop on the left where they sell wigs, hats, and comfy warm clothes for people whose bodies can't produce enough heat or keep enough hair of its own.

Pow. Sucker punch to the gut. Reality sort of slapped me upside the head. Again.

"Up to the second floor, please."

Everyone gets blood work every time they come in, so this is where my appointment began. The blood draw lab had seats lined up like a hair salon. Again with the booming business thing. The only positive was that these people were good at drawing blood. Thankfully I still had good veins (for the time being). Then it was on to see the oncologist.

He seemed nice. He explained that the results of the surgery would dictate what came next. If it was determined I was Stage II, I may or may not need to have chemo. It depended on some indicators. If I was Stage III, chemo was a definite. I already knew from reading the information on the support group what some of the factors were that determined different stages: how far into the colon wall the cancer penetrated; whether or not there was any lymph node involvement; and of course whether or not the cancer had spread to any other organs. Thankfully we'd already ruled that last one out.

During surgery, they would harvest nearby lymph nodes from my abdomen and test them to see if any cancer cells had spread to them. Since lymphs are like the super-conductors of the body, having cancer in them provides an easy way for cancer cells to "hop a ride" to other organs. This isn't a definite, but it's much more likely, so having cancer in the lymph nodes is treated more aggressively, especially if cells show up in the fluid that they use to travel in – the lymphatic super highway.

We would also hope for "clear margins." During surgery, they would remove the mass with additional areas just to the left and right. If those extra areas, or "margins" were clear of cancer cells, it would be called "clear margins." This would mean the cancer cells had not spread out from the original mass location. Basically, you know you got it all, at least at that site. Cancer cells are good hiders, so all of this is important.

Staging is a three part act: T=how far the mass has invaded into the colon wall, N=node involvement (lymph), M=metastasis to other organs. So for we already knew I was M0 (no "distant mets"). Now we just needed to know the rest.

If I did end up needing chemo, the oncologist explained, we would probably go with 5-FU. Normally there is another drug called oxaliplatin (or "oxa" for short) mixed in, but he wanted to stay away from that because oxa can cause irreversible neuropathy and I already have a pretty severe case of neuropathy (nerve damage) in both my feet thanks to a botched epidural during the birth of my son. The oncologist didn't want to risk making what I already have worse, so I would be getting just the 5-FU alone (called mono-therapy).

I was familiar with 5-FU, and knew that it could be taken intravenously or in a pill called Xeloda. When I explained I already knew those things, the oncologist asked me if I was a medical professional. I laughed. No, I was just a really well informed, kind of obsessive person who had spent a lot of time on a support group. Thankfully! Because going into this not knowing all those things would have made this visit a lot more intimidating than it already was.

Finally, he asked me if I was having pain or discomfort anywhere in my abdomen. I wasn't. If it weren't for the colonoscopy I wouldn't even know I was sick. I felt fine. In fact, I felt great. Maybe (ironically) the best I'd ever felt in my life. He pointed to a spot on my left side. This was about where the mass would be. Any pain there?

Nope. All I've ever felt were little flutters of gas. They felt almost like when a baby starts to kick.

And just like that, the idea popped into my head.

Just like a baby.

I had to name this tumor.

As you may have already guessed from the title of this chapter, the name immediately came to me: Oscar - as in the grouchy guy. He's grumpy and sometimes icky, but not really super-scary. It was the perfect name for my tumor, because I didn't want it to be super-scary. It was just a grouchy grump that I needed to get out of my can (pun intended). Then we could have a "good-bye to Oscar" party after surgery.

All in all, the appointment was intimidating but not so bad. Hopefully I wouldn't have to go back to this place too many more times.

If all went well.

Sword and Shield

Now let me explain something, because I don't want anyone to think that I'm putting on some kind of forced funny face, or trying to act as if I'm not as impacted by this as the next person. I didn't name my tumor to be phony or to pretend. I did it, literally, to make light of a grave situation. I did it so that I could face it more positively and with a laugh. In my life, I've always preferred to laugh at things rather than cry over them. Being negative doesn't usually help anyway. Being positive sometimes does. At best, my body responds to the good endorphins I send it and recovers better. At worst, I'm just happier. Not a bad trade off. There is a lot of research out there that proves staying positive really does help. That is not to say it can't be difficult to stay positive, because it can be. Especially as you face the many ups and downs that come. Things with cancer never seem to be all positive, but they aren't all negative either. It's like life, only in fast motion. The normal ups and downs just come a lot faster, and leave you feeling a little sea sick.

I don't want to let this thing define who I am. I want to kill it and have it be gone. But I also want to make the most of whatever opportunities present themselves along the way. It's part of the reason why I decided to write this all down and share it with... well, everyone.

There are so many people out there who are scared, and defeated, and hopeless. Cancer can do that like nothing else. It's one of Satan's favorite weapons, I think. Oh, you think you're tough? Life is good? You got it going on? Let's smack the old cancer stick on you and see how you handle *that*.

And let me tell you right now, I am NOT strong enough to handle it on my own. This is why I call out to God to get Satan's fingers out of my head, and his whispers out of my ears. I pray for the peace that passes all understanding, because that's what it is. I shouldn't feel peaceful facing cancer, but I do. Miraculously, I do. There is no other way for me to explain it other than to say that it's not me at all. It's Christ in me. It's His grace entirely that keeps me standing and moving forward, and that lets me carry on with hope.

The passage that I've taken up as my own comes from Psalms 3: 2-6, and it says: Many are saying of me, "God will not deliver him." But you, LORD, are a shield around me, my glory, the One who lifts my head high. I call out to the LORD, and he answers me from his holy mountain. I lie down and sleep; I wake again, because the LORD sustains me. I will not fear though tens of thousands assail me on every side."

Playing the Cancer Card

Even on the best of days, it's really easy to slip into the "poor me" mentality. I have already found myself thinking thoughts like, "I don't know how much time I have left with my child, so I'll spoil him if I want to," or "if that cop pulls me over I'll just tell him I have cancer." Oh yes, I really have had thought that. Don't laugh. It's so easy to want to play the cancer card. Over lots of things. I have to really be careful with myself and with how I relate to my husband and son. I have to be careful not to give myself too many pity parties and think that I want to be treated differently because I'm sick. Because if I were being honest with myself, I don't want to be treated like I'm sick. I don't want to be defined by this stupid disease. So if that's true, I shouldn't want to use it to my benefit, either.

That said, in spite of keeping a positive outlook, I have also found my emotions are always very near the surface. If my family has an argumentative morning, instead of just dealing with it I burst into tears. Can't help it. Once the thought strikes that life is too precious to be wasting it like this, the waterworks just come of their own free will. No stopping them.

I do realize though that this must be incredibly difficult on my husband. He is taking on the lion's share of taking care of the house and our son while I focus on recovering and staying healthy, and here I am breaking down on him all the time, or criticizing his methods. Not because I want to be critical, just because everything seems so much bigger and deeper to me right now. So while he's dealing with twice the stress, now he also has to deal with whether or not it makes me feel bad. That's a tough position to be in. I can't even imagine it. I'm aware enough to know that it's probably a LOT easier to be me than it is to be him right now. Does that mean he'd want to trade and be the one with the cancer instead? Hmm, not sure about that. But it does mean that while everyone is focused on my well-being, he's getting the short end of the stick.

I see a lot of care-giver posts on the support group that show just how stressful it can be to be the one trying to hold it all together. I've even seen people say that they don't want to know about it anymore. They wish they could put their head in the sand and not look. Not acknowledge it at all. Seeing someone you love fighting through something like this... it's devastating. It makes me realize how deep cancer really goes. It doesn't just affect a person, it affects the whole family. Friends. Acquaintances. Co-workers. Everyone.

Talk about invasive.

When I'm tempted to play the cancer card, to pity myself for what I'm going through, I try to remember these things. I try to remind myself that I'm not the only one going through this, and that I'm adding stress on those who least deserve it - the ones who love me most. The thoughts of cancer will probably never go away. The worry at finding something new and terrifying, the paranoia that every single thing you see or feel on your body might be something bad. The worm of doubt that makes you want to wonder how much time you have left to do all the things you want or need to do.

But then a more reasonable mind reasserts itself, and you know that life goes on. You can't focus on the rest. You can't dwell in it, because it can mire you down. Fear is like quicksand. It sucks at you and the more you struggle the deeper you sink.

It reminds me of my bug on a windshield story. Yes, you read that correctly.

I was going through a struggle once, praying to God to lead me and show me the way out. I was clinging to anything I could to stay afloat, scrambling around trying to find a way to get by. I knew I should let go of my fear and doubt, but I didn't know how.

I was driving one day, I don't remember where, and while I was stopped at a red light a bug landed on my windshield.

"Fly away quick little bug," I whispered.

The light changed.

"You'd better hurry."

The bug sat tight, comfortable to stay on my windshield. It had no idea my car was headed for a highway. As I turned onto it, slowly picking up speed, I watched the bug hunker down. Legs splayed, it clung more tightly to the windshield.

"You'd better go while you can," I urged it, but it didn't listen.

Its little buggy body got as close to the glass as it could, clinging to what it thought was safety. As my speed picked up, the wind buffeted the bug until it was vibrating.

"Uh oh," I worried for it, "hurry and fly before you get blown away..."

But the worse the wind got, the more it tried to stick to where it was. Finally when the speed got just so high and the wind just so strong, it couldn't keep its grip and was stripped away. It just wasn't strong enough to hold out against such force.

"If only you'd just let go when you had a chance to," I whispered, and then I realized what I'd said.

If only we just let go instead of trying so hard to hold on, to use our own strength to hold us to what we think is a safe place when the wind begins to buffet us. We have no idea that the ride we're on might hurtle us toward something too forceful for us to face. All we can do is remember to let go, and let God.

Cancer is too wild a ride to try to hold on using our own strength. It's too easy to think we can find a way to ride it out. To cling to a false sense of security, or worse, to let the fear take over. I can't play the cancer card. I have to hand it over to God, and leave myself in the strength of the everlasting arms.

Under the Knife

So next step on the cancer ride was to have surgery and get Oscar removed. I wasn't too worried about going under the knife. After all, I'm a Mom. I had a C-Section and was up and walking within hours after that. I knew from experience that getting up and walking was the best thing for your body.

Likewise, I was determined to do what I needed to do to recover well from this upcoming surgery and get home fast.

With colon surgery, getting back to normal function is the important part, so passing gas and pooping is a big deal. My surgeon warned me that she was going to come in every day and ask, "Did you poop today?"

I shared this with a friend of mine, who promptly bought me a t-shirt to wear in the hospital displaying a person with arms raised in victory and with big white letters against a black background saying, "I POOPED TODAY!" That shirt made the short list of things to pack and bring to the hospital.

I was as prepared as I could be.

I'd had my pre-op appointment that covered all the things to do to minimize chances of picking up an infection in the hospital (like washing with disinfectant wash the night before, sleeping in clean pajamas on clean bedding, washing again the next morning with the same disinfectant wash, not shaving the area near surgery within 3 days to avoid small cuts in the skin, etc. etc.). I'll admit, I didn't adhere to all of them. I can be rebellious sometimes as I'm sure you're realizing as you read more about me. Still, I felt pretty comfortable with the whole surgery routine.

It was all the rest that wasn't so easy to dismiss. Like the idea that soon we would know how deep the tumor had invaded my colon wall, and whether any lymph nodes were involved. The pathology of Oscar.

The surgery would be laparoscopic vs. open, which means small incisions to guide a scope vs. being cut open to do the resection. This is good, because healing is better and quicker. Normally surgery takes two to four hours.

The day of surgery came around, and it was time to go. I think I was pretty calm, all things considered. Mostly I remember lots of waiting, and talking silly with hubby (we like to laugh). Then it was time to go. They prepped me with something to relax me, but I do remember going into the surgery room and seeing the cool equipment they would use. Then it was nighty-night for me.

I woke up in recovery, where my body promptly tried to heave. This was about the only time I felt real pain. Dry-heaving after abdominal surgery is no fun. Fortunately this only happened a couple of times before I went back to sleep to wear off the anesthesia.

As I found out later, the surgeon told my family I'd done really well. Surgery had only taken about an hour and a half, and she felt confident we had clear margins. Nothing definite until the pathology of course, but she thought my abdomen looked good and she liked how well surgery had gone.

I don't really remember how long it was until I woke up enough to have my hubby come back to visit me, but I do remember that my throat was sore from the breathing tube (this is standard during surgery). They let me have an ice chip for that, which was heavenly at the time.

Other than waking up and the scratchy throat, the rest of my hospital stay was fairly comfortable. There were no stitches or staples. I had three small incision spots where the scopes had been inserted and one two to three inch incision just to the left side of my navel where the tumor and section of colon was removed. They used surgical glue to close the wounds. I'd read about them using super glue in the military as an emergency wound closer, and the nurse said surgical glue is about the same, just more sterile. It's a cool product, and worked very well. Plus, it didn't look nearly as grisly as staples or stitches.

I was up and walking that night - maybe eight hours after surgery. It wasn't a very long walk, but I was up! The next day I made a point to get up and walk at least three times. My pain level was maybe a three (on a scale of one to ten), and when it crept up near four I used a button to self-administer my pain meds. It lets you administer every six minutes, but thankfully I never needed that much. That first day I needed it maybe every fifteen to twenty minutes. The pain was truly not bad. More than anything it felt like having pulled muscles from doing too many ab crunches. By Friday night, I was able to put on my "I POOPED TODAY" shirt. I wore it proudly up and down the halls for my walks.

I had surgery on a Thursday, and was released on Sunday morning. It felt great to be going home, and I was glad to have had a short stay so that it wasn't too much impact on my (then) four-year-old son. The only discomfort I really felt was riding in the car when we hit bumps. The side-to-side rocking motion made me feel like Santa (belly full of jelly). I had to hold it still with my hands. Other than that and having to sleep a lot, I recovered REALLY well.

Since walking had helped so much in the hospital, and since I was out of work for a couple of weeks, I went to a local mall to do some walking. I went slow, and didn't go far, but it was great to be out. My ever-so-sweet hubby said, "Hey, there's a nice hair salon and not many people. Why don't you get your hair colored and cut and I'll pay for it?" So I not only got out, I received a wonderful makeover too.

I was able to return to work after two weeks. My surgeon would later tell me, "no one heals that quickly and goes back to work as fast as you. No one."

All in all, I had a total of about one foot of colon removed (twenty-five centimeters). The two ends on either side were sewn back together, and lymph nodes were harvested from my abdomen.

I firmly believe that it was all of the prayers I was receiving that helped me recover so easily and so soon. That, and the stubborn nature God gave me.

Pathology

After a good surgery and a quick recovery, the next step was to get the pathology from Oscar. We'd gotten good feedback from the surgeon, so we were hopeful we'd get good news, but of course we were not going to presume. Whatever was in store, God was in control.

I had an appointment with the surgeon two weeks after surgery, on a Friday, to get the results.

On Monday, I got a call that I had an appointment with the Oncologist on Tuesday.

Hmm.

When I called them back to confirm, I asked. "Is this just a follow up?"

I was assured it was. Okay. No need to worry. It was routine. But would they know the pathology results already? I didn't want to find out there. I wanted to wait until we met with the surgeon. Why? I'm not sure I can explain it. I think it's because Oncology is kind of a scary place. Not intentionally, to be sure, but still... it is what it is. And for some reason, I didn't want to learn my fate in that intimidating place. I wanted to find it out in a place that was friendlier.

It was kind of silly, really. It's not like the pathology would be any different depending on where I heard it.

So off I went to my oncology appointment. They did a post-surgery blood draw. Ah. Here, I thought, is the reason for this visit. They need to check my blood levels now that Oscar is gone. On I went to see the doc. He wanted to know how I was doing, of course, and was surprised that I was healing up so well. I proudly noted how soon I'd gone home from the hospital, and that I was heading back to work the next day. We discussed a few blood tests, and he asked me if I was meeting with the surgeon. I told him yes, on Friday.

"Well," he said, "since I'm seeing you first..." and he turned around with some paperwork in hand.

Oh crap.

Yep, there it was. Pathology results. He started to talk, but my eyes immediately scanned the page and picked up the one piece of information that seemed important. Lymph nodes 1/17.

Crap crap crap!

I knew what that meant. Cancer had been found in one of the lymph nodes.

I was Stage III.

Still better than Stage IV, of course, but...

"The tumor invaded the layer of fat on the colon wall, but that's fairly common. It's this we're worried about," his pen circled the spot my eyes had already found. "So we'll be recommending adjuvent chemo."

My eyes kept roaming. The lymph system fluid was negative for cancer cells. Well, that was good at least.

"As we discussed last appointment, we'll be doing 5-FU. No oxa, because of the neuropathy."

I was nodding along with him, but I'm not sure how much I was really hearing him anymore. I was in processing mode. I was absorbing what I'd just learned.

"There are a couple ways to administer. There's the Roswell method, which is the infusion done on site. That is done one day a week for six weeks, then nothing for two weeks, repeat process four times. Twenty-eight weeks total. Or, there's the pump. You come in, get hooked up, and go home with this pump for two days, then come back and get disconnected. We can plan to install the port..."

Port?

One of the things I was really hoping to **not** have to do was get a port. The idea of having a plug built into me so that something could get pumped into my veins just felt so invasive. Plus, going home with a pump? Really? What would my child think? What happened if he pulled on it? No no no.

"Okay, so it sounds like you're leaning toward the Rosewell method."

"What about Xeloda?" I asked. This oral method seemed so much less invasive to me.

"We've found that Americans don't absorb the Xeloda as well, so it's not as effective."

What? This totally didn't line up with everything I'd read and researched so far.

"You don't have to decide right now," he went on.

Thank goodness.

"We'll set up a chemo teach session for next week, and then go from there."

Bada bing, bada boom. I was on my way, out the door, and totally free floating. My head was spinning. This was just a follow-up. I didn't have my notebook with me. I hadn't been prepared with questions. More, now I had to figure out what to do next. Did I break this bomb to my husband on my own? Or wait and let the surgeon tell him on Friday? The idea of just popping out, "oh, by the way, found out today I'm Stage Three" seemed more than a little wrong. Not telling him I already knew also seemed wrong.

I was stuck.

I was alone.

I was going to have to have chemo.

So, I headed home. I decided not to tell hubby until Friday, when he would at least be prepared for the news. He still doesn't know I did this - he'll find out when he reads this chapter I suppose. By now we've had a chance to digest it so hopefully he won't be too mad at this choice. I was pretty mad at the Oncologist for putting me in that position, but then I thought about it and figured that with as knowledgeable and interactive as I'd been with all of the previous information, there was no reason for him to think this would be any different.

Next time I see him, we'll talk about this. From now on, he's going to need to ask me first. Do you want me to tell you now, or would you prefer to wait for a visit when you have a support person with you? That will be a requirement for any big news visits. Because finding out you're Stage III and heading for chemo without support can be rough no matter how prepared you are.

In any event, I knew right where I was headed. I needed my support group. I had tons of questions and I was no longer feeling so confident about this oncologist.

Once again, this was the best thing I could have done. I was pointed to several research studies done regarding Xeloda and 5-FU, as well as getting information on what might have constituted the odd remark about Americans not absorbing it well.

Let me interject here to say that this is an important part of your cancer and treatment journey, and something I try to share with others as I go along. The doctors can guide you, offer you their medical opinion and tell you what they think is best, but this is your life. Let me say that again. This is your life! Ultimately, the decisions about treatment are yours to make. Right or wrong. It's important to get all of the information you can, so that you can make an informed decision, and so that you can live with it. It's very easy to second-guess yourself, or to feel as though you have to do what the doctor says no matter what because they are... well, the doctor. But anyone who has been through any long-term medical treatment will likely tell you that you have to be your own advocate. You have to fight for your rights. Sometimes loud and hard. So do your homework.

I was determined to do mine.

The comment about Xeloda not being as effective as 5-FU was just flat out wrong. Several studies, including one by the mayo clinic in 2001 showed just the opposite. If anything, Xeloda was found to be more effective. As a pill that turns into 5-FU in your system, it avoids tracking through your entire body the way that the IV version does, and so targets the cancer cells with less damage to healthy cells.

In spite of that, I didn't want to just discount what he'd said. If he was right for some reason and this didn't work as well, I needed to know. I kept digging and found a couple of points that may have driven his remark.

One is that Xeloda, as a pill, comes with Folic Acid already included, whereas the IV version does not. You receive Leukovorin as part of treatment, and the amount can be adjusted. Since the 1950's, the US has added Folic Acid to several foods. For whatever reason, this has never been reversed, so many foods continue to include it (you can see it on breads, and especially in cereals as "enriched" flour or wheat flour). But while extra Folic Acid may increase the side effects, it also increases the potency, so it definitely does not make Xeloda less effective.

Another possibility is a study that PPIs (Proton Pump Inhibitors) such as Omeprazole (aka Prilosec), taken for acid reduction or reflux treatment, can reduce the body's ability to absorb things well. However, all of the studies note not to take it within two hours of taking Xeloda. Definitely do-able.

The last piece of information I found, and hopefully not the one that contributed to this doctor's recommendation, is that Xeloda is a pill and therefore the payment for it doesn't go to the practice distributing it, while the IV version does. It would really stink to think doctors would make treatment decisions based on financial gain, but it's a money-oriented world we live in. I knew that I had to be realistic and weigh this factor in, as ugly as it was.

I literally did a study on Xeloda. I wanted to know exactly what I was dealing with. In the end, my decision came down to this: I wanted to feel as normal as possible through treatment. If I could do that without compromising my own health or chance at staying alive, I was going to do it. I understood the likelihood that certain specific side effects might be slightly higher with Xeloda, namely the hand and foot syndrome. This is where the smaller capillaries in your palms and on the soles of your feet tend to store up the toxicity from the chemo, which can dry them out and cause redness, pain and skin peeling. There are ways to mitigate this, such as slathering cream on your hands and feet every morning and night. Drinking lots of water helps, as does getting exercise to help keep blood flowing to extremities.

What else affected my decision? Work. I am the one who carries our health insurance, so staying employed was very important. While my workplace and boss had both been extraordinarily supportive so far, taking three to four hours a day once a week for twenty-eight weeks would add up. Eventually my sick, vacation and FMLA time would be used up. What happened if I then need time off because I just felt crappy? Got an infection? Or, God forbid, ended up in the hospital?

I had to put my health first, but if I lost my insurance, we could not afford Cobra on one income. Maybe I could get fast-tracked on SSDI, but in the weeks in between I'd either be without treatment, or racking up a crap-load of debt. That wouldn't be good for my health either. Plus, if Xeloda didn't work out, I could always switch to something else. Done deal.

My decision was made.

With this small amount of control back, I started to finally settle and make peace with what was about to be my future.

Six months of chemo.

The Good with the Bad

On Friday, as planned, we met with the Surgeon and hubby received the news I'd already gotten.

There was some new information. Even without the lymph involvement, I would still have been recommended for chemo based on how far the tumor had penetrated the colon wall. I had not realized this. Or maybe the Oncologist said it and I was just too dazed to take it in.

On the good side, I was healing extraordinarily well. I had been back to work for two half days and one almost full day, and was feeling great. Plus, partly thanks to hubby's salon treatment day, I looked great. The surgeon told us, "No one heals this fast and is back to work in two weeks. No one." She was very hopeful that given how healthy I was and how well I did with surgery, I would be able to handle the chemo without too much trouble also.

Leaving that appointment, on the way out the door, I said something that later came back for deeper discussion.

Because what faced us next was breaking the news to all our family and friends, all the people praying for me and sending their love, that we had good news and bad. What I said was that I felt like I'd somehow let them down. Yes, it was great I was healing so fast, and great that there was no sign of cancer in the lymph system, and if you have to have lymph involvement, one out of seventeen was the best we could hope for. But it still meant Stage III, and it still meant chemo.

Later, on another night talking to my husband, I tried to explain that feeling of having let people down somehow. I wanted to talk about it to him, and I want to talk about it here in the book because it's a very real, very pervasive feeling.

It's as though if I don't try hard enough, or stay positive enough, or handle everything well enough, that I'll have somehow let everyone down. Like if I have cancer, it's somehow my own fault for not fighting hard enough and I'll have let my family down. It's not all completely rational, but it's there, that feeling. Like if I don't have enough faith, I'll let down everyone praying for me.

To help explain it, I likened it to me being a star basketball player, and everyone coming to a game to support me, to cheer me on and wish for me to win the contest... and then to lose. I would have let all those fans down.

To me, this analogy was one I hadn't put into words until that night, but it so well captured my feelings that I became emotional. It's so wonderful to have support. So many people don't. And it's so wonderful to have my faith, and know that I have so many prayers coming from so many people and places. It still doesn't stop my human heart from wanting to make good for those people. To be the miracle story. To prove that there's hope.

Like I said, it's not all completely rational. The truth of the matter is it's not curing the cancer that proves there's hope, it's the face of hope as I go. It's not whether I am cured for life or not, it's how I live with whatever time I have.

I said something in the description of this book that I want to explain. It says, "I'm determined to be a survivor. Even if it kills me." What I mean by that is, even if cancer eventually claims my life, I want to have not just had the disease; I want to have lived well throughout. I want to have kept my joy, and shared my heart, and continued to help others in any way I could with every single moment that I have. In that way, I will have "survived" no matter what the outcome or longevity of my life is.

Chemo Journal - Week 1 Part 1

<u>T-1</u>

I start chemo tomorrow.

I shouldn't be nervous, but I am. It could be a breeze, it could be awful. No one really knows. It could be that I don't have many side effects at all, but that the cancer comes back. I could put my body through all of this for nothing. The bummer is I won't know for months. Or years.

<u>Day 1</u>

I was so nervous last night I was fluttering around like a bird. Hubby (bless him) gave me a back rub that helped me fall asleep. Taking the pills this morning, knowing I was willingly swallowing something that is poison was super-freaky. All the horror stories of what can happen during chemo start to take on a really terrifying reality when you're getting ready to down the stuff. Could I really lose teeth? Could my feet and hands turn black? Will I have painful mouth sores? Will I lose my taste buds? Have first bite syndrome? Become allergic to a food I enjoy? Get infections anywhere bacteria can hide? Get dizzy while driving? Ack! Sheesh, okay. No wonder I was nervous. Chemo is crazy scary stuff. They should name it something less frightening, like FLUFFYPUFF!

(Yeah, *there's* the old Tracy! I knew she'd make it back)

I got onto the support group today. I needed it. I was worried about the dosage they'd given me. It seemed super high. I called the oncology pharmacy to verify. They were very nice, and glad I called with this kind of question. They rechecked that it was filled as prescribed, then rechecked that the prescription matched my chart, then actually recalculated my weight/height to dosage ratio and verified it was good. That made me feel better. Being on the support group and reading through more Stage III survivor stories helped too.

It's just after lunch, and so far so good. Not really feeling anything other than the after-effects (and probably ongoing a little) of nerves. I have decided that I want to switch myself from Omeprazole (PPI inhibitor style acid reducer) to Tagamet aka Cimetidine (H2 blocker style acid reducer). This is a little against what the nurse practitioner suggested, as she thought it might add to any stomach upset, but I feel strongly about it as there are studies showing Cimetidine may actually help fight colon cancer by not allowing cancer cells to adhere to the colon wall. In my opinion, that makes changing worth it. Not to mention I've wanted to get away from Omeprazole if at all possible. Long term side effects are just beginning to be known, and I suspect they'll find more. Anyway, an okay Day 1 overall.

Onward!

<u>Day 2</u>

Paranoia sets in. Every boo-boo or pain results in a moment of... "Is that the chemo? Am I having side-effects?" Arghh. I know that if and when they do hit, I'll probably know it, but it's hard not to second guess. I also have to be careful not to baby myself. I want to keep life as normal as possible, but it's easy to start to fall into that "I can't do that, I'm on chemo," or "treat me this way, I'm on chemo." It's a pity party waiting to happen is what it is. So easy to fall into. I sometimes think that when Satan finds he can't get into my head with fear, he tries self-pity as an alternate. I'm sure there are other pitfalls as well that he will wave in front of me as I go. Overall, I still feel really good. So for now I am going to hold on to that. I've placed all this on the altar; I'm going to leave it there.

Chemo Journal - Week 1 Part 2

<u>Day 3</u>

Weekends are hard. In order to maintain the same medication schedule I have to wake up early, eat something, wait a bit, take meds, go back to bed. Without thinking about it too much, if possible. It's hard to sleep after pumping yourself full of poison, just on a mental level. The day went by okay, although I ended up wiped out and needing a nap. I can't really say if that's due to the chemo or just being the mom of a five-year-old.

We visited some friends we haven't seen in a while, and I had to ask myself - are you going to tell them about the cancer or no? Telling them seems almost like asking for pity or something, but not telling them leaves a lot of questions like why are you so tired when you haven't really done anything? Yep, it's true, cancer seeps into EVERY corner of your life.

Day 4

This day started out a little rocky. Did the weekend morning routine, but found myself feeling mildly nauseous when I got up. This lasted for about four hours. Wasn't bad enough to make me unable to eat, and I didn't actually get sick, it was more a feeling that simmered in the background. Sort of like being sea sick. If you've ever been, you may be able to identify when I say you think being sea sick will be a feeling in your stomach, but it's actually more a feeling in your head. Sort of like being dizzy without anything spinning. It leaves you feeling off kilter and nauseous. This was similar to that. I didn't really have the urge to be ill; it just sort of left me off kilter. Just enough to know it was there.

Midday I went shopping then took our son to Grandma's for a family birthday party for him, and was feeling a bit better after walking around a bit. It was nice to get to visit and feel fairly normal for a while, if a little wiped out. Went home and needed another small nap.

By nighttime I began to wonder if the nausea was from the chemo, or my change in acid reducer meds. Could be either, I guess. So now I'm torn between whether I should keep on and just tough it out, or go back to the original meds and risk the chemo not being as effective. I suppose I should consult the doctor.

Day 5

Didn't feel like getting up today, but I have the feeling that staying in bed would only make me feel like staying in bed more, if you know what I mean. Is giving in to this feeling of tiredness and emotional overload what makes the "side effects" really take hold? Do people just get too exhausted to keep feeling positive, and the rest creeps in? I also wonder, if this is only round one, what are the next few months going to be like? I think forcing myself to get up and get going is probably a good idea.

I definitely have some acid reflux going on, but I think I can get through it. I'll definitely talk it over with the doc(s) to be sure they are at least aware. Few sore spots in the mouth, although I can't see any actual sores. I am trying to brush every time I take the meds, to be sure it's not the direct contact that is causing that. It may also have to do with the acid in my stomach. Nothing too bad, overall, just stuff to keep an eye on. Think I'll risk the folic increase and eat some crackers to soak up the excess tummy acid.

I'm finding that as of last night / this morning I feel a little more emotional than usual. Old Satan trying to get me down when I'm in a low spot. I listened to my gospel music this morning, and heard one song that said "hold on, keep going" and another that said "God is with you even when you're at your lowest." I pictured him like a parent, worried about a sick child, and of course burst into tears on the highway while driving. I feel like I'm pregnant. Hormone overload (or maybe just overwhelmed). Funny all the things that go through your head.

<u>Day 6</u>

What a difference a day makes. I do wonder whether chemo messes with hormone levels. I'll have to ask the doctor that. The Lord is definitely sending me some messages through music. I woke up this morning with a song stuck in my head. It's called "Don't Start Doubting Now" by the Dunaways, and the lyrics talk about not letting fear and worry rob you of your joy.

How true that is. If you have a chance, go listen to the song or find the lyrics. They say it better than I can.

When God Spoke to Me

So, I have a funny story I had to interject here. One of the lines from the song of encouragement that God gave me that I talked about in the last chapter – "Don't Start Doubting Now" by the Dunaways - says "God understands the words you're not saying; don't question if he hears the praying." And it struck me that sometimes when you're going through something like this, you stop and realize that life has gotten away from you and you haven't prayed in a while, or as often as you should have. But the reassurance that I feel those words give is that even when you're not formally praying, you are still talking with God. He still hears you, even when it's just a stray thought or random moment where you call out to him.

I have confidence in this because of an experience I had when God spoke to me.

I used to work in a very stressful environment, not only because of the work itself, but because of some of the difficult personalities I worked with. I had taken to saying a prayer before every meeting to be sure I had His help with my words, thoughts and actions. Without it, I often felt like I was heading to a firing squad.

So there was one meeting that I went to (I can't recall now the specifics of what it was about, but I remember I was nervous about it) that went pretty well. I headed back to my office with a smile on my face, and as I stepped through the door the thought hit me. I forgot to say a prayer before I went! "Oh Lord," I whispered, "I'm so sorry I forgot."

And very distinctly, I heard these words in my head. "*I didn't.*"

They were so quick in response, and not something I was thinking at all, that a thrill raced through me. I knew without question that I had just heard the loving voice of my Heavenly Father reassuring me.

There's a song I particularly love that is about a woman with Alzheimer's. It's a favorite of mine, because a very dear friend of mine ended up with this wretched disease. She has since gone home to be with God, but this song and these words always make me think of her. It's sung by Archie Watkins, and it says, "Should the day come when I can't remember Him, He will remember me." These words of hope are applicable to Alzheimer's, but also I think to general life. When we commit to Him and make him our Savior, it's not just about remembering to pray at certain moments. We're always talking to Him, in everything we do throughout our lives. So should a day come when I don't remember Him, I can be confident that He still remembers me.

Chemo Journal - Week 2

<u>Week 2 Notes (random)</u>

I ended up doing some research to find out whether chemo can cause hormone imbalance. I was going to pose the question to my support group, but the answer came up everywhere, so it was pretty evident that it does. I suppose it makes sense, because taking hormones can cause cancer, so it would be logical to then think that treatments to eradicate cancer would also affect hormone levels.

I think this particular side effect is easy to overlook, as having your emotions close to the surface seems pretty normal for someone facing cancer anyway, and then there's the depression aspect also. For me, it's when the emotional response starts to feel out of proportion to the cause that I start to think it's more hormonal.

As it turns out, having chemo can also bring on menopause.

Oh, and this weekend I found out that having chemo can also cause you to lose your fingerprints. Yep, lose 'em. Mostly that's due to hand and foot syndrome, and the tissue damage that it can cause in some cases, but apparently if you are being security checked in an airport and for any reason they need to check your fingerprints, if they can't get a print they ask whether you have had any medications such as chemo. Interesting factoid, eh?

Personally, I'm still feeling pretty well overall. A little more tired than normal, some heartburn that won't quit, and here and there a little hormone overload. If that's all I have to deal with during the next twenty-six weeks, I think I can handle that. It could be much worse. Maybe I wouldn't have said that a year ago, but I can sure as heck say it now.

End of Week 2

Hooray! My week off starts tomorrow! I'm so happy to get a week off. Even though side-effects weren't all that bad, it's hard to describe how happy I am to have this break.

Start of Off Week

Misconception - I will immediately feel one hundred percent better as soon as I have a day without chemo.

Reality - still more fatigued than I would be, still not helping out as much as I want to be with mom duties and house work. I suppose by the weekend I may be feeling a little stronger, and I can volunteer to help out more. That way I can stop feeling so guilty that I'm not doing much to help.

Oncology Revisit

The good news is, my blood levels are looking good! My iron counts are coming up, my liver functions look good... excellent!

The bad news is, my blood levels are looking good, which means I'm okay to fill my chemo prescription at the same dose. Not that that's bad news, it's just... well... not exciting. Checking off one more three week cycle (two weeks on, one week off) is nice. Eight cycles total, one down, seven to go. Try not to get overwhelmed. Try not to think about your odds of a recurrence, or what that would mean in terms of being a *lifelong* chemo recipient. Definitely don't think about what happens if it doesn't work and you end up Stage IV (which as someone eloquently put it today means "no hope of a cure." - Gee, thanks for that).

Yeah, it can get you down, going to Oncology. Even for good visits.

God knew that. As I pulled into the parking space, the song on the radio was "Hold on to that last thread of hope."

Thanks, God. I needed that. You always know!

Give and Take

Had an interesting conversation with the woman who provides social services at the Oncology clinic today. We talked about support (and how blessed I am to have it), and about needing to take care of one's self during this time. As I started thinking about writing a chapter on the topic of taking care of one's self, it struck me that there aren't a lot of words to correctly summarize it, at least not well.

Selfish of course, carries connotations of being greedy. The dictionary phrases it as being "chiefly concerned with one's own interest or advantage to the total exclusion of the interests of others."

Huh.

So how does one characterize the need to pay attention to your own needs without this negative perspective?

Well, I thought, normally as a wife and mother I am a caregiver. So in this case, I am needing to be a care *taker*. Only, those words don't fit either.

Caregiver (according to the dictionary) is defined as "a person who cares for someone..." while

Caretaker is similarly defined as "a person who takes care of another."

Double huh.

So, how do I say that I need to focus on taking care of myself and putting my own health first, without saying I'm doing so at the exclusion of the interests of others? More, how do I *do* that? I can let people know what is happening, share with them my trials, let them know I'll be focusing on getting well... but how do you really put yourself first when your very role in life is to put others first?

As I'm finding out, it's definitely easier said than done. Lots of people say, "if you need anything, just let me know!" However, when you are exhausted at the end of a relatively uneventful morning, and need to call someone to entertain your extremely active five-year-old for a while, those volunteers become scarce or otherwise engaged pretty quickly.

When we first had our son, we could laugh this off. Yep, people promise a lot of things they can't deliver. The road to hell is paved with good intentions, and all that. We could almost laugh it off, or at least shrug it off. Dealing with the same thing while handling cancer and subsequent treatment is a lot different. Now we don't just want help, we *need* it. Not just for the stuff others might think of, like hugs (although those are good too), but for good old fashioned work.

This comes to light for me now, during me "off" week, because I found myself immediately feeling guilty for not picking up more slack around the house for my poor, exhausted hubby. Instead, as I learned, just because you are a day without the chemo does not mean you immediately feel great and full of energy. It might be day two, three, or even four before that happens, if it happens at all! Only way to know is to test it out and see what "trends." That doesn't help poor hubby, which only makes me feel guiltier. It's an off week! Suck it up, woman! Plus, hubby tries to do everything for me, and winds up spending all his energy being both of us.

My support needs support!

And here's an important additional point - as the social service woman pointed out rather eloquently, you shouldn't have to spend the only time you have feeling really well catching up on housework and running yourself ragged. You need to enjoy it and use it as a time to re-energize in prep for the next round. Man, she's right!

So how do I do this?

What I've realized is that I need to change my entire mindset. I need to not be afraid to put people's noses out of joint. I need to be persistent. I need to be a pain in the butt. I need to let people know not to offer unless they mean it, because I *am* going to take them up on it. I need to become kind of a bully. At the very least, a tougher version of me. The key, at least in my mind, is to accept that this is not because I am excluding the interests of others, or putting myself ahead of my family. It's because I need to do this in order to be there for my family in the long haul. This is a marathon not a sprint, as they say.

By learning to take what I need in order to get where I need to be, I actually give to my family. By taking time for me, I can give more of myself to others. Seems simple, but take a look sometime and see how often you really do this. How often do you say no to the boss, because you really do need time to regenerate in order to remain a good, healthy employee? How often do you say no to family because you really do need an afternoon just with yourself or your spouse?

It's quite an interesting perspective, but one I think I will learn a lot more about over the next several months.

Chemo Journal - Round 2 Part 1

Heading into the next round of chemo was a little daunting, but not overwhelming. Days one and two usually go by fairly unchanged. Days three and four are when the fatigue usually hits. And the emotions. Or maybe it's just the reality of it slapping you in the face a little. I watched an episode of a show where a girl had cervical cancer. She was bald, but shopping for a wedding dress. She and her fiancé had decided to get married as a celebration of the end of her chemo. She was pretty in spite of her lack of hair, and very happy, brave and strong. She got married on a beach. At the end of the show they flashed a message.

In loving memory...

Oh God.

She was only twenty-four.

There aren't a lot of happy endings when it comes to cancer. That's the stark reality of it. There are short roads and long roads, but you can't wait for the "ever after." The happiness has to happen along the way. I suppose that's true of life in general. Sometimes we're just more aware of it. We must live each moment. I know that I won't die today, or tomorrow, or the day after that. I don't know whether surviving this chemo will be the end of my cancer story or if there will be more chapters. Sometimes facing the reality of a possible future, or lack of one, is overwhelming. That's when I have to cling to my faith. To the promises that are there for me.

Because the reality is that in the end, that's all we really have to hold on to.

Faith.

Love.

Hope.

Chemo Journal - Round 2 Part 2

Well, here we are into week two of round two. Another off week on the horizon and then one more round will be under the bridge. I had a follow-up appointment with my surgeon yesterday. She walked in and said, "Well you're here by yourself, you're driving, you're working, all while on chemo... you're amazing."

I was confused for a moment. "Should I not be driving?"

"Well a lot of people can't. A lot of people can't work, either. Of course some people breeze right through it, but I was afraid I would walk in here and you would say you felt sick, your hair wasn't shiny, it had turned curly--

"Wait!" I shouted, hands to head with a giant grin. "My hair could actually turn curly?!?"

Since most people reading this have never seen or met me, allow me to explain. I was bald until I was two. As a little girl, my mother had to tape bows to my head. My hair is so straight and so fine that most barrettes just fall right out.

They don't even hold. UGH. Dozens of perms later, I am still endlessly jealous of those with naturally curly hair.

At this point, doc laughs at me. "Yes, it's been known to happen."

Now, let's temper this conversation with some reality. She did mention a lot of people start to feel the side effects in rounds three and four, which are still ahead. I've heard some folks say they were fine until round seven, and then things got really rough. So there's just no way to know how one's body will adjust, and even if things are good now, how they will be in the future. I know this.

But let's add a dose of good news, shall we?

I now don't need to see my surgeon again for three months, at which time we should have a good handle on how chemo is really going. She was also happy I had changed to Cimetidine (instead of Omeprazole). Every little thing could only help.

"If we can keep you cancer free through year five, that's the magic number."

Deep breath.

Now for those of you who don't pick up on subtleties let me say it more plainly: As of right now, I'm considered cancer free. Surgery removed the tumor, I had clear margins, all my numbers are coming back up. There is **N**o **E**vidence of **D**isease (aka "NED" – you'll hear me talk more about this later).

The key, of course, is to keep it that way. But I'm going to focus on that "cancer free" phrase.

Because sometimes, you just have to grab it and run.

ISOMELTED

You may be wondering whether or not it ever really gets to me. Do I break down?

Yep. Last night was a major meltdown. I **so** melted down (hence the chapter title).

On June ninth, I started round three out of eight of my chemo. I also turned forty-seven. Happy Birthday. My family has been asking me what I wanted to do for my birthday this year. I didn't really feel the need to celebrate. That's more for little kids. Just something quiet and nice is fine. No need to make a big deal. Honestly, that's as far as my thoughts had gone on the matter. At least, that's what I thought at the time. Sometimes the human psyche can really surprise you.

So last night, Junior had a rough night getting ready for bed, which is always tough because I hate yelling at him, but sometimes it still happens. At some point, he realized he was supposed to be good because it was Mommy's birthday the next day. When your five-year-old asks you what you want for your birthday, the first thing that comes to mind should not have to be: *To be able to see you grow up. To live to see my next birthday, and the next one after that.*

I don't like to cry in front of my son, but there was just no stopping the deluge that ensued. He hugged me, and said, "Now go get a tissue and wipe your face." Normally this would be cute enough to shake me out of it, but not this time. I couldn't stop. I managed to get him to bed, and then went to have a good cry. Anything and everything that had been building up rolled out. When hubby came up to check on me, I told him I was 'getting a grip.' What I was really doing was purging. Letting loose. Of course, some of the things I was letting out I hadn't even known had crept up on me, but they did.

Things like the odds. All I seem to hear and see lately, are stories about people who are famous for their spirit, the way they can overcome anything in life and the way they have joy no matter what. How everyone expects them to conquer illness the same way they have conquered everything else in life. Only they didn't. Somehow, the miserable sour people are the ones who live on, while the gentle, joyful souls are the ones who have to battle things like cancer and live on only in 'loving memory' stories. I told my husband, "I don't want to be a story." It makes you start to think that maybe if you are a miserable wretch, you somehow have better odds at surviving.

But after my meltdown, as I finally started to breathe normally again, something struck me.

You say the word Satan, and somehow your words start to come off like science fiction. Even people who believe in God can have a hard time talking about Satan like the real thing. I believe completely that he is real. I also think I've threatened him. When I dared to be a joyful person, he decided to toss cancer at me. See how I'd take that one. When my joy and faith not only went on, they became stronger, I think he was mad. But when I started sharing it with others... well I think that made him absolutely furious. I think he's been dropping these images in my lap. You want to live? Try out being miserable instead of joyful. Try doubting instead of trusting.

Sneaky, manipulative creature.

Even this morning, as I was listening to songs on the radio about how in the dark times it's hard to remember that Jesus Loves You, I was in that fragile emotional state.

I didn't want to celebrate sucky cancer birthday.

What I do want to celebrate is all the other birthdays that will come after this one. Satan's attempt to steal my joy may have required a cry session and some deep breaths, but I have God, and His grace will always be greater.

Today, I'm forty-seven, and no matter what Satan tries to throw in my way, whether it's cancer, or doubt, or sadness, I am going to keep shining my light. That's who I am. That's who God made me.

Round the Bend

So here I am in the middle of Round four out of eight. Almost half way done! My thought was that I would wait for more eventful things to happen before writing the next chapter, but I'm finding that people are interested in knowing where my mind and body are at, so it was time to resume.

Round three was mostly uneventful. I did end up having a bit of hand/foot syndrome. Mostly it's in my feet. They have little dark spots showing up all over. I describe it as that they look moldy. Sometimes they have a darker red cast on the toes, ball and around the edges of the heel, but it's hard to tell what's normal red and what's "syndrome" red. Near the end of Round three, they started to feel "blistery." By that I mean that it felt as if I'd worn new shoes and had blisters, and was walking on them. However, if I looked, there were no actual blisters. Just the feeling. I called the docs and they had me stop my chemo a day early (no biggie). I continued to slather on lots of lotions, and tried to bump up my fluid intake. This helps flush the chemo residue out. Within a couple of days they were feeling a lot better.

For Round four, they decided to decrease my dosage very slightly. My concern, of course, was that this would decrease the effectiveness, but I learned something new. Apparently when they have patients that are more susceptible to side effects, such as elderly or already medically fragile or compromised, they do the dosage in reverse. They start at the lowest possible dose, and gradually increase until they reach the point where they're at the max the patient can handle. So for me to start at the max dose for my body mass index (BMI) and gradually decrease if needed, I will not necessarily decrease the effectiveness of my treatment.

Another option we may consider is the regimen that does one week on, one week off vs. what I'm doing now, which is two weeks on, one week off. This supposedly has similar effectiveness, but allows the body more "off time" during treatments to allow the body to recuperate.

The important thing is to keep managing myself effectively. I know the heat just wilts me, so I work with the lights off, the blinds drawn, the AC up and a fan on. I try to minimize my time outside and in the sun to nearly nothing. Kind of sucks not to be outside when it's nice, but I'm not good with heat anyway, so for me this isn't a big sacrifice.

Now that I'm at the end of week one in Round four, I'm noticing the foot blistery feeling coming back a bit. So today I'll be pumping fluids as much as I can.

An interesting thing to talk about is the hand part of this syndrome. For the most part, all I've noticed is that sometimes my fingertips look a little darker than normal. I wonder if I will have the issue that some others have mentioned, and will lose my fingerprints. I suppose I could become a cat burglar, and spend my life stealing cats from unsuspecting owners, but then I'd be up to my ears in litter, so... nope. Seriously though, the folks on the support group have joked about this. You have to joke about it. You have to laugh. There's no other way to handle the myriad of strange and funky things that cancer and chemo can bring you.

Anyway, I find myself studying my hands and fingers much more closely than I ever have before. I feel as though I know them more intimately as a result.

The only other thing that's happened to me since last we spoke is that my life has taken a bit of a turn. Don't worry, it's a good turn. I've mentioned before that I look at this experience as an opportunity. Since my diagnosis in March (just four months ago), I have completed a book (that I had previously been working on for over a year), am over forty thousand words into book two in the series, am fifteen thousand words into *this* book, and completed a short story spin off of my series that is just over eight thousand words. So I have written somewhere in the neighborhood of one hundred and twenty-five thousand words in those four short months. To what can I attribute this burst of productivity?

Let's be honest - it was finding out that I had cancer. It galvanized me in a way that nothing else ever has. Not that I want to have had it happen this way, but once I found out, I knew I needed to finish the book. I couldn't consider that I might die without ever having completed it. No one else knows my characters the way I do. No one else knows what I want to have happen, or how. It became my focus to complete my story. So while this wasn't the way I wanted it to happen, I surely can say that I have hit my stride because of it.

The really good news? On July second, the short story I wrote was accepted for publication. The people that work with this particular publication are not only huge names in the Fantasy book world, they are also writers that I love and have great respect for. My goal was really just to get my work in front of them. To find out that they liked it enough to want to publish it? That was pure icing on the cake. As of October or December of this year, I will officially be a published author.

Wow. Saying *that* is pretty awesome.

I used this as an opportunity to query the Literary Agent who was at the top of my list, and am crossing my fingers that I might convince her to represent me. Also, Book Two in my Series made the final round in a writing contest and because of that is being read by an editor at a publishing house who works with Fantasy. That's pretty awesome too.

Maybe by the end of my chemo and cancer journey, I will be able to say that 2016 was both the worst and the best year of my life. God certainly has his hands on me, steering me on a path of grace and glory.

Be Your Own Advocate

I've heard those words so often that I sort of feel as though they've lost all meaning. I hear so many scary medical stories. People who are misdiagnosed, or not diagnosed at all. People whose doctors make them feel as if it's they're fault they're sick, or worse, that it's only in their heads. When dealing with something as big as cancer, being your own advocate takes on a whole other level of proportion.

Let me try to explain. One of the stories from my support group was from someone who was told, right before Christmas by the way, that there was nothing more that could be done. They were beyond hope. They should gather family, call hospice and prepare for the end. Can you imagine?

The support group then led this to another drug, which was one of the newer ones at the time. Two months later, this

Stage IV person has achieved Disease Free Status (or "DFS"). No evidence of disease (or "NED").

Another story - one of the people I've become close to on the support group is now being told there are too many liver mets, and that the meds aren't working. She was given three choices. Keep going as is and knowing nothing is going to get better, stop meds and just live it out, or go with a radical and very risky surgery that might provide good results... if you live. Wow. Some choices. After many tears with her family, she shared this with the support group. Results? She was promptly invited to France where there is a doctor who very successfully performs this surgery, and where other Stage IV patients have achieved CURE. That's right, CURE.

From hopelessness to hope purely based on who you are talking to.

My own experience comes to this also. Somewhere around the beginning of round five, I presented my oncologist with the suggestion of changing to the one week on, one week off regimen. To show him I'd done my homework and wasn't just spouting off, I provided two studies that showed this might be beneficial. The studies looked at various regimens and compared effectiveness and side effects. The conclusion they came to was that Xeloda (and 5-FU) reach maximum effectiveness at day eight and that everything after that (within the regimen) increases side-effects without providing additional benefit.

Since most of my "blistery feet" symptoms began on or around day eight, I thought this was a fabulous idea. However, I didn't want to ease my symptoms if it meant lowering my chances. These studies seemed to prove it wouldn't. So I suggested it.

My oncologist turned me down flat. He said: "That regimen is not indicated for curative."

Really? My first question was, "Is it *contra*-indicated?" Which means, do studies show it's less effective at achieving a cure, or are they just not on the bandwagon yet?

His overall answer to me ended up being that while in ten years this may be the standard, it's not yet, and he doesn't want to deviate from standard.

Hmmm.

Not what I wanted to hear.

Some weeks later, I would discuss this point of view with another wonderful doctor while my dad was in the hospital (he's an epileptic, so I kind of grew up in hospitals). She noted, and I agree fully with her, that any doctor going into oncology as a profession isn't doing it to be a bad guy. They want to help. The problem is I live in a small town. Small towns are not on the cutting edge of medical treatment. I shared with her that I had sent an e-mail to a rather prominent oncologist known for his treatment of GI cancers, and he was willing to consult my case. However, by the time I got my medical records sent down and heard back from the hospital, I was already mid-way through round 6. I decided to finish my treatment, but any future needs for oncology will mean a new doctor.

My oncologist is not a bad guy. However, I don't want my future in the hands of someone who refuses to treat the individual, and is only willing to stick to what he knows as a standard of care. I've learned that it's not good enough.

The doctor I was speaking to about this agreed. She told me point blank, "if it ever comes back or spreads, leave. Get out of here. Go to New York City, or Boston, but don't stay here."

I think it's good advice, and something I need to be adamant about, because no one is going to fight for your life harder than you are. You have to trust your gut, and fight back, and push boundaries. Be your own advocate takes on a whole new level of meaning. At the very least, don't take no for an answer. Is there anything left we can do? No. --Time to find a new doctor.

Surviving Cancer

Wow! It's already September. October and the end of the Chemo Road is just around the corner. Now that we're nearing the end of this portion of the journey, I feel a little better giving perspective.

So what has it been like?

Well, like everything else in life, it's had some ups and downs. Just after I finished the last chapter (which would have been a couple of months ago now), I read in my support group about someone who had finally lost her battle with this wretched disease. To honor her, I went back to read some of her posts so that I could get a feel for who she was. What I read really tore at my heart.

Her last post was titled, "When do you tell your kids that you're going to die?" Punches you in the gut, doesn't it? But it's a very real, very necessary conversation for many of us, even those of us who aren't at that point yet. Why? Because how our families are impacted by this, especially our children, is probably foremost on the minds of those going through it. As a Mom, I would rather go through it than have my husband or son suffer. I'd gladly bear it in their place a thousand times over it meant sparing them. However, sparing them from losing me is something I have no control over. It's hard, not having control. I know I have to leave that in God's hands. What I *can* control is my message to my family that comes from how I live my life, how I face trials and even how I approach the subject of death.

I think, and many of those on my support group feel the same, that not telling your kids that you are sick and might die can be more traumatic than telling them. Especially if something does happen.

I think the more honest and open I am, the easier it will be if and when my son has to face something like that. However, I'm careful to tell him that it's not something we're expecting to happen anytime soon. We're fighting the good fight against Mommy's "bad cells."

Still, no amount of self-realization or rationalization can soften the blow of that topic. It affected me for quite some time. I couldn't write about it at first. It was just too raw, too sensitive of a topic. And okay, yeah, a little scary. How do you admit to someone else you might die when you don't even want to admit it to yourself? It's a lot. Just that - it's a lot. I cannot emphasize enough how absolutely blessed I am to have a loving family, an amazing husband, and a God that gives me his strength when mine is just not enough. If you want to know how I can get through something like this, how I can face those terrible questions and what-may be's, that's how. I'm not strong enough. Not even close. Not on my own. Thankfully, I'm not on my own.

Another result of a cancer diagnosis is that everything that happens to you afterwards, every ache and pain and fever, jumps immediately to cancer in your head. Before my diagnosis, I might have thought, "Gee, what if this is cancer?" but then my mind would immediately answer itself with:

"Don't be paranoid. You're fine." After diagnosis, that check and balance is gone. Now it's just... "Has it spread? Has it come back?" You can't tell yourself that it's just senseless worry, because it's not. Having had cancer increases your chance to have it again, and to have other kinds. Cancer really sucks that way. I have ovarian cysts. My chances of them developing into cancer go up because of having had colon cancer. So any pelvic or lower abdominal pain is going to lead to worry.

I'd love to say that with as close as my relationship with God has become over the course of my life and this journey with cancer that I don't worry, but that would not be truthful. I'd love to say that I give it all to God and that's the end of it, but that would be a lie. I do worry. I do fret, probably more than I should. The difference is that it's not my whole life. It's a moment here and there. Like one of my favorite songs by the Crist Family, "It's just a feeling that comes and goes - my head may doubt, but my heart knows."

Now let's talk about the good stuff.

I went to my follow-up visit with my surgeon, and she said to me, "So, you drove yourself here, you're still working full time, you've written two books, are working on another one, have gotten published, and you're a Mom of a five-year-old?"

I had the grace to kind of blush. She called me a Rock Star. Yep, capital letters and all. I don't feel like a rock star, but hearing it all summed up like that makes me feel good about what I've managed to do. It's sort of like hearing God say, "Well done, child." You just have to glow a little.

So here I am, nearing the end of my six month journey with chemo. For the most part, life has continued as normal. Money is a little tighter, my energy is a little lower, but God is carrying us just as he always has and always will. What's next? Lots of follow-up exams, plenty of doctor visits and blood draws, a CT scan here and there, etc. etc.

Five years NED is the magic number. Once you make it five years, your chances of recurrence go way down. Between now and then, I just keep living and keep the faith. Every memory I get to share with my family is a blessing. It always was - I just realize it a lot more now.

My husband and I went to a church service this last Saturday night, and the minister was talking about Jesus healing the blind man. He read from John 9, verses 1-12, but it was verses 1-3 that really struck me.

John 9

[1]As he went along, he saw a man blind from birth. [2] His disciples asked him, "Rabbi, who sinned, this man or his parents, that he was born blind?"

[3] "Neither this man nor his parents sinned," said Jesus, "but this happened so that the works of God might be displayed in him."

When I was first diagnosed, I asked the surgeon if I should change my diet and lifestyle. Did I cause this? She reassured me that I did not cause my cancer. "Plenty of people with poor diets and lifestyle never get cancer." Conversely, plenty of people with great diets and very healthy lifestyles still do.

Call it bad luck, or genetics, or just the fate of this old world. People are quick to think things, to assign reasons why bad things happen. It helps them to deal with it better than thinking it might be random and out of their control.

I don't think it's my fault I had cancer. It's not my parents' fault either.

For a while, my mother felt guilty because she prayed for me to come closer to God. She wondered if my cancer was an answer to that prayer. I ask her, "Would you give me cancer to teach me that lesson?" Of course, her answer is an emphatic no. "Neither," I tell her, "would our Heavenly Father."

So who sinned that I have had cancer?

No one.

It's not my fault, nor my parents fault.

I wonder then, did my cancer happen so that the works of God might be displayed in me?

We all wonder why bad things happen. Why God allows them to. I've always believed that God knows the outcome of life at such a level that we cannot begin to understand, but every once in a while, we get a glimpse. I've always said that my motto is that "If I can help somebody as I walk along, than my living shall not be in vain." This is my chance to do that.

I don't believe that it's God's fault people get cancer, but I do believe he can use it for his glory if we have faith. We can be a light in the darkness with our words and our strength, and even by just surviving, because life is a gift.

So this is my prayer.

Whatever the future holds for me, I hope that this, my journey, shines a light for others. That I am able to give someone hope by having hope. That I can let someone know they can survive, by surviving.

Even if it kills me.

Because surviving isn't about living so much as it's about how you live. I'm going to live my life, every second of it that I am given, in the light.

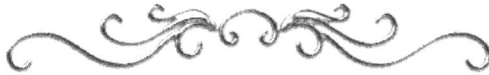

Words of Encouragement

The posts below are words of encouragement and feedback that I received from others while writing this book. The fact that so many of them were themselves touched by cancer or a devastating illness just showed me the reality of how many suffering hearts there are out there, and the power that words hold, especially when filled with the Holy Spirit. Here are a few I wanted to share. Thank you to those who posted them for not just the encouragement, but for allowing me to share them along with my story. God bless and keep you all.

I agree about honesty being the best in these tough situations. I always told Jesse the truth, even when I had to tell him he would die. Hardest thing I ever did. I struggled with that later, still sometimes wonder. But not a whole bunch because I had decided that my boys would hear the truth from their dad no matter how sad or uncomfortable. It builds trust.

I pray that your cancer journey will be over and that you will have many fine years with your family. But of course, I don't really know what will happen. I do know that you have been given grace from our Heavenly Father to face this and whatever else comes your way. You are a child of the King and that is always an adventure. -- Peter Wiebe

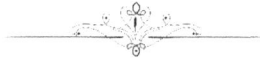

Tracy, right from the first time I saw your face on WO (Write On) I knew you were special, but, hey, I didn't know you were a sister in Christ and also a sister in colon cancer. Wow. Mine was Stage I, but should never have gotten that far. Did so due to me ignoring my

doctor's suggestions I get a colonoscopy. Finally after 9

years I did.

I love the personality with which you write. I loved it

so much it seemed I read your posting in six seconds flat.

No way. Really. But truly seemed it. Please keep writing.

I love your statement of magic. I believe with you it is a

God given magic.

THANK YOU FOR SHARING YOUR MAGIC WITH ME!

-- Warmly and with xxoo Muriel

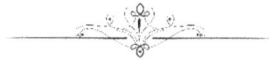

I'm praying for ya and a cure. I'm a cancer family

survivor. My mom had lung cancer, by brother-in-law has

lung cancer, my 1 & only cousin has breast cancer, my

grandson's mom has liver cancer, my dad HAD colon

cancer and he has been cancer free for about 15 yrs now.

You are an awesome writer and God has definitely

given you some great insight to use your gifts. Keep it

coming. It's like the Living Water it has to flow and your ministering words are flowing out of you and into many someone(s) that need hope.

And remember we're not only readers, out here, but we're prayer warriors too. – TEW

Stories from other Survivors

Before I end this book, I'd like to share some stories from some of the other folks on my support group. They have inspired me, lifted me, helped me, and given me my power back. At the bottom there is information about this person's individual cancer information. This is how the people in the support group see what others have, what they've taken, how far along they are, etc. at a glance. These stories are in their own words.

God has given me the chance to share my words, spread my light and find freedom. I want to share that magic with my friends. You'll see them only as the handle or online name they have chosen. I see them as much more. They are my comrades in arms.

My fellow Survivors.

cptmac

It was on July 22, 2004, my 43rd birthday, that I heard those words, "you have Stage IV colon cancer, you have 6 months to live, but you could die at any minute." I was so angry, that I wanted to live 6 months and a day, just to prove that doctor wrong. I never could have realized then that I'd set my sights way too low...

Let me tell you a little about myself back then. I had moved in May of 2003 to a new state for a job. Previously, I'd always had a full time job, been in the reserves and freelanced, so I didn't have many opportunities for philanthropic work. But when I took this job it was the only thing I was doing. After living in my new state for a year I felt confident in my position, but a little bored. I prayed to the Lord that whatever he needed me to do, I had time to do it. I would let him pick my path. I would let him pick my work for charity.

At the same time, I needed to renew my prescription for my allergies. I stopped into a walk-in clinic for a prescription for them. The doctor stated it was probably allergies, but suggested I get a colonoscopy to rule out IBS or Chron's disease. Not to worry; it wasn't like I had cancer or anything. So I did some research on IBS and Chron's and made an appointment at a different facility with another doctor who tried to talk me out of it. He said I was too young, I had no symptoms, my insurance wouldn't pay for it and he informed me that walk-in doctors aren't the best physicians. However, I had done my prep work and a friend and I had taken the day off of work, so I went ahead with the procedure. He asked me to come back on Monday for the results.

When I saw him, he stated I was lucky that I chose to have a colonoscopy. He had found something. He went through the stages of cancer. He said they would know more once my biopsy was back. His statistics (at the time) indicated that only five percent of people survive Stage IV cancer and, on average, individuals usually only lived for eighteen months after diagnoses. Feeling as good as I did, I thought, even if it was cancer, it obviously was in the early stages, since I didn't have any symptoms. I purchased a lot of books and scoured the internet and felt assured that I was fine, since I didn't have the symptoms.

People say that they will never forget the day that they found out that they had cancer. For me, it will always be easy, it was my 43rd birthday. I then went to yet another facility to meet a colo-rectal surgeon. He confirmed that I had Stage IV cancer. He told me that I had six months to live, but that I could die at any minute. He seemed nice at first, until I told him that I would be getting a second opinion. He glared at me, and I knew that I would never step foot in his office again. He became angry with me and informed me that he would not have time to talk to me about the surgery, but he did let me know how dire my situation was. I needed to plan the surgery ASAP. That even with treatment I would live for 18 months tops, but that I could die at any moment.

He proceeded to let me know the excruciating pain that I would be in when my colon burst and my gastric juices would flow throughout my body. That I should not fly on a plane, that I should not lift anything, that I should not eat anything, because these could make my colon rupture.

I held my ground and stated I wanted my medical records so that I could take them with me. Well, he didn't have them, so I had to retrace my steps, going back to the different medical facilities to pick them up in a city I barely knew. None of the places that had my records would release them without me personally picking them up.

I remembered the words of that doctor, the excruciating pain I would be in. I thought, how would I get to a hospital? Perhaps suicide would be better than the pain. I thought about running right into a concrete median. But thought, what if I killed someone else, and that doctor had made a mistake? How could I live with myself? I thought about driving off a bridge, but what if I broke my legs, and it turned out not to be cancer. I thought about OD'ing on drugs, but didn't know what prescription drugs would do it. Then, out of nowhere, a car tried to pass me on the shoulder and hit me. Now, not only did my odds seem hopeless, I was also transportation-less and over fifty miles from home, with a cell phone that was dying and all my friends calling me up and wishing me a happy birthday. Telling people I was about to die could wait until after my birthday.

You would think I would have known better. Cumulatively, I've had some of the worst birthdays. It started with my folks forgetting my birthday when I was seven, and continued through my life when I had to go to court on my birthday to have a family member who had Alzheimer's put in an assisted living facility against her will, and on, and on, and on…. Whenever tragedies happen in my life, I try and figure out what life lesson I'm supposed to learn. Seeing a doctor on my birthday I should have known not to expect anything good. Okay, I did buy a lottery ticket; after all, wouldn't that make a great headline: Woman dying of cancer wins $22 million dollars, has six months to spend it. So WHAT LESSON WAS I SUPPOSED TO LEARN????

And then I knew. I knew, because once I admitted it, it was the first time I started to cry. I was always a giver and was too independent, too selfish, to ask for help. Even then, my independence made it difficult for me to ask for it. I thought about my next step and who I would call. After all, I'd barely known my coworkers for one year. I picked up my phone and called a co-worker to pick me up. I called someone who I thought could keep a secret. I let them know the dire nature of my situation because I still needed to pick up my records and I had time to do it, but I knew he was a bit of a lollygagger. I asked him to not tell anyone. I got a call back that he couldn't pick me up right away, however, another co-worker's brother lived right by where I was. He was a stay at home dad. He would pick me up and help me get my records. What??? Now another co-worker knows??? AARRRGGGHHHH. My lesson would be hard learned.

Well, his brother had a hard time finding me, and none of my

records could be picked up because it was after five o'clock by the

time we met each other. He drove 45 miles-an-hour on a 65 mile-

an-hour highway to get me home. I wanted to strangle him, but

it's true what they say, it's far harder on the caregivers than it is

on the patient. All I wanted to do was go home. I was having a

horrible birthday, and the sooner I went to sleep, the sooner my

birthday would be over. Tomorrow would be a better day.

Tomorrow *had* to be a better day.

Every year, the week of my birthday, US News publishes its list

of best hospitals (you can find it

here: http://health.usnews.com/best-

hospitals/rankings/cancer). I set up appointments at the

University of Minnesota, the Mayo Clinic, MD Anderson Cancer

Center. My birthday was on a Thursday. The University of

Minnesota made room for me on Monday, Mayo on Wednesday, MD Anderson on Friday.

The first thing I did on Friday was read my horoscope. It said as long as I saw a doctor early in the month, everything would be okay. I went to the walk-in clinic on July First. Yay!!! I was elated. This was the first bit of good news I heard. It gave me the motivation to continue. My co-worker gave me print outs that our administrative assistant printed out of airline flights to Minnesota. *Great, now she knows too.* I made my airline appointment, called friends to take me to the airport, meet me at the airport, etc, etc. I now knew the importance of not seeing doctors alone. I emptied out my fridge, gave food to my neighbors, bought a lot of cat food to feed the stray cats I fed, then I started to pack. I filled two suitcases with all of my worldly belongings. I packed my Bible, my prayer Bible, my rosary, and several books about colon cancer. I kept looking and laughing, as I had no clothes in the bags. But then I thought, I'm going to Minnesota, the home of the Mall.

Clothes would be easy to find. I wound up taking every thing that was important to me, that would be irreplaceable. I know now what I would take if I ever needed to leave my home in an emergency.

I looked around my place thinking, "I may never come back here again." I took photographs in my brain of what I had and what I'd accomplished. The next day someone was there to take me to the airport. There was a torrential rainstorm, but I had a nice friend who picked me up and carried my suitcases to her vehicle and to the plane. After all, if I picked them up, I could die. She never complained once.

On arrival at the University of Minnesota I found out that they too couldn't get my medical records. I was forced to redo all of my tests. Turned out to be a great thing, because they had newer CT scan equipment. Their pictures looked a lot better and were electronic. All of my doctors and tests were within walking distance. No more getting lost and trying to find my way around.

After my results came in, I met with my oncologist, Dr. Edward Greeno. All of the other doctors spoke highly of him, and let me know that he would be the mastermind behind my whole journey. Not only did he give me hope, he gave me options. He let me feel that I could have some control throughout this whole process.

One of the things that we talked about was a Phase II clinical trial. I remembered trials from a Statistics course I took in college. I understood the years of research it would take before a trial could be offered to patients. I also understood the different types of studies that needed to take place before drugs could be cleared through the FDA (Food and Drug Administration). Katie Couric's husband's doctor had just published a book right before I was diagnosed. Talk about lucky me. In it, he talked about the use of an HAI pump. This interested me. Well, the clinical trial that was being offered to me involved the HAI pump. Talk about lucky fate.

I've always been a supporter for the advancement of science and I knew I would never have a problem signing up for a Phase III clinical trial. However, Phase I and II trials frightened me. I was sure that only the sickest of the sick would sign up for those. Then I realized, I *was* the sickest of the sick. Doctor Greeno explained everything to me in great detail and gave me the forms from the trial to read. He gave me a lot of confidence in helping me understand what was involved. I appreciated all of the research that had taken place before I even started the trial and all of the safety issues that would be put in place to ensure that no harm would be done to me.

I've always been concerned that I would become addicted to drugs. I interrogated all of the medical personnel whenever I was given a new drug. One time, after my liver surgery, they wanted to give me a sleeping pill, because I was awake almost all night, and I needed a good night's rest for all the tests I would need the next day. The conversation was about ten to twenty minutes long, until someone said the common name of Benadryl. Heck, I take Benadryl for my allergies. they should have started with that info.

A few weeks after I was released from the hospital from my liver surgery, I was still feeling a bit of pain in my abdomen. I was weaning myself (not doctor ordered) from my pain meds. I had an appointment on Monday and would get a refill then.

Doctor Greeno had an ultrasound done of my abdomen just in case. When a friend took me to pick up my prescription at Walgreen's, I saw, for the very first time in my life, a white squirrel. I took that as a sign that everything would be okay. It was a good thing too. My friend and I went shopping and got some groceries. We watched some TV and then I checked my voice mail at eleven PM. In ever increasing urgency were seven voice mails. The first four were from my nurse; the last three were from my doc. I needed to return to the hospital immediately.

Upon entering, I was told to put on a gown and lay in bed. I wanted to know why first, so we had to wait for the doctor. He ran in, wondering why it took me so long to get there. I am fidgety and talk with my hands. He kept telling me to stop moving. I could tell he was stressed. I thought perhaps because I woke him from bed. As I kept moving he kept telling me to stop and to lie in bed. He finally blurted out "You have a blood clot by your hepatic artery!" Okay, I've heard blood clots are bad. But my appointment was at two PM. I'd gone shopping, climbed three flights of stairs up, and then down again. I didn't understand. And then he yelled, "Don't you get it? If you don't stop moving, you are going to die!" I stopped, and he walked out of the room, I think to regain his composure. I asked my friend and the nurse to leave so I could change. But I would be moving…. The doctor talked to my friend outside, who was in shock. This was the first time he heard that I could die imminently. I had never seen him so upset. Once I was in bed, I asked if I could move my arms and legs, or was it just my torso that I couldn't move? He frustratedly said "Arm, yes. Legs, barely" At that, since I am quite the walker, they supposedly lost my clothes until the day I was able to check out. I think they did it to make sure I didn't escape. That wasn't the first time it happened to me, but it cracked me up that they thought that I wouldn't leave the hospital in my stylish gown. Since I hadn't packed at all, my friend bought some books for me to read. It's nice to have great friends. It's nice to ask for help.

At this time, the Terry Shiavo case was all over the news and I started wondering about my own fate. Would the rest of my life be filled with endless doctor's appointments until I was finally sent home one last time to die? I was becoming annoyed because I had not started chemo, and I felt my journey's end slipping further away. Even more so, because it's hard for me to sit still, much less lie still. All that changed when doctor Greeno visited me in the hospital and assured me that the worst was almost over. I also remembered that I'd seen that white squirrel. It gave me hope.

What was even scarier, once I started chemo, I started losing my personality. My handwriting got very small and neat. I started talking slower, I started typing slower, I started walking slower, I barely slept as I constantly wanted to walk. This happened over the course of two weeks. I didn't want to say anything. After all, who complains that their handwriting is now neat and small? I mean, they are going to send me to the loony bin. I have similar handwriting as my father, and when he was ill, his handwriting looked smaller, but not as small as mine. I was concerned that I would be put away forever. When I couldn't sit still for my appointment with doctor Greeno, he sent me to see a neurologist. They did an MRI (magnetic resonance imaging) scan of my brain. The residents were VERY impressed on my sinuses and complimented me on them. I almost started to laugh. I asked, "Does this have anything to do with what's wrong with me?" They said they really didn't know how to read the report, but they didn't see anything. I then saw the neurologist, who wasn't sure what was wrong with me, but said he would send my info to the head neurologist. He informed me that this guy is the same guy who ultimately decided Terry Shiavo's case. I became really nervous. I felt as though my fate was about to be handed to me. That there was no hope left. After all, if he got to decide Terry Shiavo's case, would anyone take me on if he gave me no hope? Thank goodness he called back within five minutes. My body was reacting to the Reglan I had been given with chemo to alleviate nausea and stomach upset. Apparently, I'm one of the very few people in the world with which Reglan causes medically induced Parkinson's. The neurologist showed me the symptoms from a poster he had on his wall. Sure enough, your handwriting becomes very small and neat, you talk slower, you walk slower... All the symptoms were there. Now, whenever I go to a doctor's office, I read all the literature. You never know if you might be able to help your doctor diagnose you.

Once, while I was getting chemo, I was wondering if signing up for a clinical trial was such a good idea. And then, in an instant, came a crawl on CNN. Patients who sign up for clinical trials do better than patients who don't. What???? Surely I'm delusional.

Did I see that right? Luckily, my chemo took an hour and a half, so I had time to sit and watch it crawl by again. Sure enough, there it was. I never doubted my treatment again. I never doubted that God sends you signs when you need them most. Luckily, I've never needed a sign since.

My oncologist really helped me through it. He never made me feel that he didn't have time for me. I always felt that I was his priority. This may not seem like such an amazing feat, unless you understand how I tick. Example: At my appointment with doctor Greeno toward the end of my treatment, which was at four in the afternoon, I'd come prepared. I had a list of things to go over with him. There were over a hundred questions on my list. I figured I would just keep asking until he shooed me away like so many other doctors. Okay, partway through he did mention, "it looks like you have a lot of questions there." I said, "Yes I do, so I hope you're comfortable," and kept asking questions. But doctor Greeno stayed until after five o'clock and never once looked at his watch or seemed annoyed. I knew he would help calm my fears of my cancer returning, because I now knew the reason so many people are scared of cancer. You don't even know you have it.

What makes Dr. Greeno a great doctor is, he explained everything to me in a manner in which I could understand and was not the least bit concerned that I was tape-recording every word he said. Not only did he make me more knowledgeable, I have been able to pass on this knowledge to other patients who are too timid to talk to their doctors. Several of them thought they were incurable, and I convinced them to get another opinion. Several of them have now been told they can be cured.

Due to doctor Greeno's patience with me, as I gained knowledge about my disease, I have also used this information to enlightened friends of mine who were both State and US Senators. If not for doctor Greeno's tireless efforts of answering my questions and keeping me informed, I wouldn't have the information for them to help others.

People will ask if you've changed from having cancer, I say not really. I've always been a very positive person, but I have learned some valuable lessons.

1. I'm excited because I've already had the worst day of my life. I can't imagine any day being worse than that. And, it was the worst birthday of my life to boot. Some people will say, what about the day you die? Heck, I'll be dead.

2. When you first move to a city, find great hospitals and doctors first, not where the best stores are.

3. My life has gotten easier now that I have learned to ask people for help. It makes them feel valued, and I'm able to get a lot more things accomplished in my life. I used to think I needed to learn everything, now I say let the experts who know Excel, do Excel for me. And if I google things I need in an Excel program, chances are, there is an Excel program out there for me, for free even. I

found a checkbook program, medical bill tracker and one for taxes. That is really all I need.

4.   The most important thing I've learned is, God has better things to do than to find me a hobby.

Thank you for letting me share my story with you. I share it every year, because when I was diagnosed, I was looking for any Stage IV's who had survived. Message boards were not what they are today, and I couldn't find anyone. Now, thanks to the message board that I belong to,

(http://coloncancersupport.colonclub.com) I have found many. Thank you to everyone on support group(s) for sharing your stories and for helping the newly diagnosed find their way through this maze.

I hope you'll share a smile with me, to celebrate my birthday/cancerversary. I no longer dread getting old, I am thrilled that I am alive!!! I am so blessed to have so many friends who are willing to help me and celebrate my birthday with me!!! Thanks

for letting me share!!!

--cptmac

"As long as you're alive, there is hope."
Diagnosed 7/2004 stage IV
colon resection 8/2004
liver resection 9/2004 with HAI pump installed
Phase II trial with irinotecan as systemic and FUDR for
direct chemo to liver via HAI pump
Cured since 9/2004

Lee's Story

I was 46-years-old and going through the change of life when my hemorrhoids really started to act up. I'd had little issues with them most of my life, but now not only were they itchy, I was also seeing some blood when I wiped. It was about six months later I finally mentioned something to my primary care doctor about it. He confirmed my hemorrhoids were indeed bleeding. Since I was due for some blood testing because of other medical issues he decided to add a few other tests that should have been a red flag for colon cancer. All my tests came back negative or normal.

My doctor also wrote a referral for me to get a colonoscopy. Those bleeding hemorrhoids were going to be my excuse for getting my baseline colonoscopy early in life. He said, "call them today because it will be while to get in." Yep, just to see the GI (gastro-intestinal) doc took three months. GI doc was not worried about finding anything. No history of colon cancer on either side of my family. My mother had her first colonoscopy at fifty-five and found no polyps. My dad had died early in his life

(Vietnam war), but none of his relatives had it. On the way out the

door, the nurse had just hung up with a patient that had canceled

their colonoscopy scheduled for that Friday. I had first dibs if I

wanted it. Sure let's do it and get this behind me. No pun

intended.

I prepped with horse pills that I had to take with lots of

water (never again -- I'm not sure if they even use them anymore,

I know I won't). In the morning, a friend dropped me off while my

dear husband got the kids off to school. I remember during the

procedure the doctor saying he had just found cancer. Afterward

in recovery with my husband, the doctor said he'd found a

tumor. It was small, less than five centimeters, probably stage I.

Surgery for sure, maybe some light chemo. We would talk again

next week one the pathology reports came back.

Over the weekend, I decided not to wait. I called the

doctor's office Monday morning and the nurse scheduled me to meet with an oncologist and surgeon within a few days. I saw an Oncologist the next day. She was the first person to give me a hug and say it's going to be okay. That hug went a long ways toward make me feel better about my situation. She set me up with a radiologist.

The next day I saw the surgeon. She scheduled me for a more in-depth procedure. During that procedure she took a sample of the tumor and found 4 lymph nodes were affected (surgery would confirm 6 nodes positive for cancer). She also found that the tumor had grown through colon wall and was wrapped around my colon, now 8 X 11 centimeters. I went from Stage I to stage III rectal cancer. We told the kids that night about my cancer. They were nine and eleven years old at the time. A week later I started radiation. Radiation was the worst for me. Destroyed 2/3 of my rectal muscles early on, thus I was tied to the toilet anytime time I ate. Most days I did not eat anything until I knew I was home for the day. Not a way to live your life.

Saw my surgeon after radiation and she sent me to see a wound/ostomy nurse. This is where I learned about a colostomy. As my husband put it, you have options, but mostly you can get your life back after cancer. I knew I wanted that colostomy bag and called my surgeon the next day. Told her she could take as much as she wanted, just get all the cancer. She said I was making the right decision. I had the surgery on a Monday morning and I was up walking those halls by late afternoon. Four people went with me that first walk. I was doing solos by the next day, and I walked, walked, walked those halls. I was finally released Friday night.

Seven weeks later, I started chemo. At that time, FOLFOX was experimental, had not been approved by the FDA and was only available to stage IV folks. But my Oncologist knew it was coming and chose me to be her first patient due to my youth and overall good health. She got me on board with a trail group. I took my first dose in my left hand, as my Oncologist had to fight my insurance company to get approval for a port. They were so new, most nurses did not know how to use them. I had my port for my second dose of FOLFOX. I was three months into chemo when the FDA approved FOLFOX for stage III and stage IV folks only. Avastin was the other new drug to come out. These two drugs would increase survival odds when dealing with colon cancer.

I was one of the few people who actually gained weight while on chemo, but per my Oncologist I was not allowed to lose even a pound until I was three-and-a-half years out from diagnoses. Even then it was to come off slowly, no rapid weight loss (thus I joined Weight Watcher's and am still a member today). When I finished chemo, I started power-walking. I was a couple of years post diagnoses, when AMA was advising cancer patients to exercise, as this could reduce chances of a recurrence by up to fifty percent. At that time I was walking three times weekly, for about thirty minutes. Today I still walk for about an hour three to five times weekly.

Finishing chemo is exciting and scary at the same time. You are so excited to be finished, yet scared because you no longer feel like you are actively fighting your cancer. Maintenance is a scary time also, like waiting for the other shoe to fall. Appointments, scans and blood tests every three months, then every six months, than yearly. You try to live your life as best you can between appointments. I was four-and-a-half years out when my Oncologist made a comment about dropping me at the five year mark. I left her office with tears in my eyes. Tears streaming down my face when passing the waiting area. Uncontrollable sobbing inside my car. For the first time since my diagnoses, I knew I had beat my cancer.

I continued to see my Oncologist for a few more years. She would close her office and I was forwarded to a new Oncologist. Last years I was told I was CURED, it was not coming back this far out (eleven years). Words I thought I would never hear. I don't see an Oncologist anymore, and while I still think about it almost daily, it does not consume me like it used to.

While life goes on, life is not the same. Life gets back to normal, but it's a new normal. You can't go back to the person you were prior to diagnoses. I carry in my heart many people who did not make it. I am so grateful to all the doctors, family members and friends who helped me on this journey. It is because of all these people I am very much alive today.

--Lee

rectal cancer - April 2004
46 yrs old at diagnoses
stage III C - 6 out of 13 lymph nodes positive
radiation - 6 weeks
surgery - August 2004/hernia repair 2014
permanent colostomy
chemo - FOLFOX
No Evidence of Disease ("NED") - 10 years and counting!

Miss Molly

I had to add this section after reading a particularly poignant post by our own Miss Molly. While it deals with some of the more difficult parts of the cancer journey, I found it extremely touching and insightful. In it, she is responding to someone who has a close friend who is suffering from a lot of pain, and a prognosis that is not very pleasant. If you are a friend or someone wanting to provide support for someone going through this, I think you'll find it amazing. Thank you, Miss Molly, for giving me the okay to include this in my book.

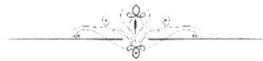

As someone myself who is on the final length of life after years of fragile health and also occupying a body riddled with pain, I offer that you take a less energetic approach with your friend.

For any person facing a life-threatening illness, there can come a point where there seem to exist two realities: The reality and day-to-day life of those who are healthy and the reality and day-to-day life of the one who is gravely unwell.

I describe this inflection point using the analogy of driving down a interstate freeway. The healthy bodied continue down the interstate at 60 mph, a straight plane trajectory. In my illness, I have had to take a detour exit off of the interstate, a curved bypass at a reduced speed of 15 mph to a destination unknown.

Your friend may be feeling this change in her reality in facing her diagnosis, therapies, and horizon of an uncertain pelvic exteneration. Your friend may be feeling as through she has taken an exit ramp while you continue with life down the interstate freeway.

Another way of looking at the life of a person with serious illness is through the lens of a football game. Spectators and players engaged and enthralled in the excitement of the game. On the sideline, sits the person with serious/life-changing illness. Life continues on seemingly without interruption. It is a surreal feeling, as the person with a life-threatening illness is now a passive observer and less an active participant. The emotional impact is one of deep isolation, a deep divide.

Unrelenting pain is an experience that can only fully be acknowledge by those who experience it. This is pain that has no end point and no reprieve. Although my pain cannot be seen on the outside, it fills every fiber of my being and every neuron in my brain - it is all consuming. Narcotic medication lowers the volume of my pain experience but does not remove it. Narcotic medication allows me a space of time where pain moves from all consuming to a sustain nuisance. I am on a hefty narcotic cocktail of Fentanyl and dilaudid, enough to knock out a herd of zebra. And, yet, pain racks my body.

That said, I urge you to approach your friend with a softer presence. Although you mean well with your encouraging rallies of a "girl's night out" when she is recovered, you are not tapping into your friend's true needs.

Your friend's true needs are more a focus on support in this immediate moment and less on support in the distant horizon - which may be a horizon that she can barely discern. Your friend's lack of a smile when you mention "girl's night out" is a polite non-verbal expression to you that she doubts of her future to be able to attend to such an event. My advice: Meet your friend's immediate emotional and physical needs.

What do I want most from friends and family who visit and interact with me?

A calm, quiet, and comforting presence. Because of the pain that I experience, even conversation with another person is added noise. Be respectful and offer a calm and quiet presence when conversing with your friend. Be comforting in your words and actions. A touch of a hand, a gentle and sustained hug, even a foot massage - each add an element of human connection.

I do not appreciate boisterous visits where friends regale to me of their week's adventures and upcoming plans and activities. Can they not see that I have difficulty even standing and walking to the bathroom, while they are telling me about their upcoming trip skiing on Mt. Hood.

Offer to read a poem or book with your friend. I have one friend who comes to visit me and each visit she reads a chapter of book. I have limited attention to read as I did before, and I appreciate her being a personal audio-book. She is attentive to keeping her voice quiet and to observing me if I am uncomfortable or if we need to stop.

I appreciate small gifts wrapped in tissue paper. A pair of fuzzy socks. An adult coloring book with brightly colored pencils. A tube of lightly scented body lotion. A basket of assorted herbal teas and a ceramic mug. A pair of cozy pajamas. A few assorted, popular magazines.

I appreciate a car ride. Riding aimlessly around the city, just to get out. Riding to a city park. Riding to the Reed College campus. It is important to get fresh air and a change of scenery for one's mental health.

Personally, I do not want gifts of food. The colliding smells of foods can be un-welcomed.

I do appreciate it if people pick up for themselves as they leave a visit with me. If I have a few dishes in the sink, I appreciate it if friends and family will take the time to wash and dry the few dirty dishes. I appreciate people helping me with managing my paperwork and organizing my bills, as my attention span is less than it used to be.

Most of all . . . a calm, quiet, and comforting presence.

Most of all . . . a listening presence. I appreciate friends and family who will listen to what I need to express, even if the topic is uncomfortable for them to listen to and process. There can be a profound sharing between friends when faced with serious illness.

Do not be afraid of real conversation. Do not divert a conversation by saying, "Oh, let's not talk about this. You will be just fine."

Serious/life-threatening illness is a personally isolating experience. Sitting with visiting friends, I can feel particularly lonely. How is this, you ask? The isolation comes from the innate experience that my life's reality is no longer that of my friends and family that surround me. Be sensitive to this dissonance that your friend may be experiencing.

Being a true and trusted friend to your friend's immediate personal emotional and physical needs is the greatest gift that you can offer. Your friend is inviting you into her life at a difficult crossroads. The shared experience between the both of you is as real as it gets if approached with sensitivity and care.

--Miss Molly

Devoted daughter to my father, age 80, diagnosed with stage 2 colon cancer Nov-14
Dear friend to Bella Piazza, former CC member. Prayers always to Bella.
I, myself, have a permanent ileostomy and sometimes offer advice on living with a stoma/ostomy.

I have been on Palliative Care for broad endocrine failure + Addison's disease + osteonecrosis of both hips and jaw + immunosuppression with recurrent infections for 3 years, recently transitioned to Hospice Sept-16. I am A-OK with my decision.

BeansMama

I'm very pleased to be able to add this chapter. One of the people on the support group that I've mentioned at various times in this book recently gave me the okay to include her story. Following are a series of posts that will walk you through her journey from her first post to one of her most recent. Like me, she's a Mom, so we share some perspective on being "Mom Warriors" through this journey. I hope you will find her story as encouraging and brave as I do. We call her BeansMama.

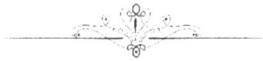

INTRO POST - Jan 2016

Just wanted to say hi and introduce myself.

I started to write out my whole story and realized holy crud it was long, so the cliff notes version it is.

My diagnosis is stage IV Colorectal cancer. I have metastasis to my liver (one large tumor that is actually beginning to grow out of my liver and several spots) and had 4 lymph nodes come up positive.

Napkin ring tumor found in September 2015. Insurance issues forced a wait until November.

1st surgery, sigmoid and a good portion of my rectum removed. Proud owner of a spanking new colostomy. But had the hope it could be reversed. Had issues with a weird discharge, opened incision site (tumor in the sigmoid was too large to remove laproscopically) and placed a wound vac

Home from hospital for 3 days before doing my impression of evil knevil. Felt a pop but it didn't hurt so I kind of blew it off. The next morning everything went to hell. It involved an incision filled with stool and a super fun ambulance ride with my incision only covered with gauze.

2nd admission, 2nd surgery. Lost more colon, colostomy moved and now permanent. I now have the wound vac placed on 2 sites. It was determined the original colostomy was breaking down causing the weird discharge to begin with.

Weeks of healing, vac dressing changes, a rectal abcess and sepsis. I would really prefer to never be admitted to a hospital again.

Finally get to start chemo next week. Can only do Folfox for now because my wounds have not healed fully. The plan is to add Avastin when the wounds are healed fully.

I can honestly say I'm scared. It's hard to hear your oncologist tell you that he can't say you will be cured. I keep thinking I'm not done yet. I have a family that I want more time with. I know the Dr. has to be cautious, and I know I will fight like hell to beat this but it still weighs on my mind. Hence posting this at 1:30 am...

Anyway, that is the long / short version of my story. I look forward to getting to know people on here and sharing support as we all travel this journey.

⁓

Back in the chapter of this book called "Life Changer," I mentioned a post that turned my perspective completely around. That message came to me from none other than BeansMama. Following is that post.

Tracy,

I totally understand searching for information and trying not to obsess about it. But the simple fact is you will obsess about it. Even now, when I know what I am facing I obsess about it.

I worry constantly about how my illness affects my daughter. I try to keep things as normal as possible but the sad fact is things have had to change. I have had so many complications she's used to seeing me in the hospital, she's had to become more of a helper at home, she does like being on "mom duty" because she feels like she is in charge of me though. It bothers me that she has had to grow up pretty fast in the last few months, but I try to think of it in a positive way. She's learning that we help family and others when they need it and that with determination we can do anything we put our minds to. She's seen me overcome a lot already, and I have promised her that I'm not going to die so I better try my hardest and then some to beat this.

Things don't always go as I have planned - and that planning nature of mine gets me in trouble with this disease. It's one of the reasons I research and obsess and try to find new or different treatments.

I wish I could tell you it goes away or gets easier, but at least for me it hasn't and I'm not sure it ever will.

Don't lose confidence in future scans, I have found PET scans are pretty dang accurate, and it all depends on who is reading the scan. Some doctors are better at it than others. I have had I think 7 or 8 CT scans since that first one (I have lost count!) the others with better interpretations. I also think knowing what is there helps them interpret other areas of the scan.

***

Of many difficult things Beans has had to face on her journey, one interesting twist was having to move during treatment. This meant, among other things, a change in doctors. Following is her post about her first appointment in her new locale.

The appointment went very well!! He wants to treat this very aggressively, he is going to follow through with the stump issue too! I get to see a GI that will scope me again but will use a scope that not only has a camera but ultrasound as well so they can get a better picture of what is going on in there.

Got some awesome news, he said it looks like the small tumor in my liver is "dead". It shows up as calcified on the last CT scan I had and it did not light up in the last PET scan.

The big tumor is another story. It stopped shrinking. It is half the size it was originally which is good but the Folfox was just keeping it stable. I will be switched to folfiri with vectibix starting next week.

I am feeling very positive about this and I think this was the right move for us.

Anyone have any info on folfiri and vectibix? I like to be prepared for what may happen. I know he did say I was basically guaranteed to get the rash that goes along with it but they will be able to manage it.

UPDATE Sept 2016

Saw the onc, according to him. He has not seen the vectibix rash get as bad as mine was after the first treatment. Gave me oral antibiotics that I will be on for the duration to see if that helps. His nurse gave me some lotion samples to try for the lizard skin.

I do have a funny, someone entered my pharmacy into the computers incorrectly. My script was sent to a pharmacy in a completely different state!

I haven't been on much lately, I have really been struggling the last week or so. It has been an emotional roller coaster to say the least.

I have the full blown vectibix rash. I feel so ugly. I rarely leave the house (only if I absolutely have to) and it hurts! My skin is not only red, bumpy, has more pimples than a kid heading to their Jr prom, and itchy, but it hurts like hell too.

I am also heading into what I refer to as the lizard phase. It is becoming dry and scaly on top of everything listed above. I have resorted to organic coconut oil with some soothing essential oils that also combat infection mixed in. Regular lotion just was not doing enough. The catch 22? Scales better, pimples worse.... Oh and I'm shiny...

Thank God hubs loves me unconditionally because I know I have been a bear to deal with this last week on top of everything else he has going on.

Anyway, thanks for reading my whine fest. Anyone have any idea of there is a light at the end of the vectibix tunnel? Or will I deal with this the entire time I am being treated?

THE HARD UPDATE - You all also heard me mention in Be Your Own Advocate chapter, someone who received 3 options, none of them great. Thankfully, on the support group, you receive more than just sympathy. You get advice, usually from others who have gone through the same. The person I noted in that chapter was also Beans (yep, she comes up a lot in my journey), and following is her post about this very difficult next part of her journey.

So, had treatment 16 today, the plan is to use the compazine until disconnect day, I will get an IV of fluids at disconnect and start taking steroids for three days following disconnect to see if it works for the nausea. The next option is the cannabis pill if that doesn't work.

Saw my onc obviously. I have three options that hubs and I have to discuss. 1) Keep doing what we are doing and I get 2 more years. According to the oncologist. 2) We can fight the insurance and try and get me on immunotherapy drugs to keep me stable / can't guarantee a cure for however long they work. 3) Surgery. The thing is I may not survive. They would take my liver out of my body, rebuild my abdominal vascular system, remove all the tumor from the liver and basically reconstruct it, then put it back in. It would actually be more than one surgery as they would have to force the left side of my liver to grow in order to ensure they have enough liver to put back. According to my onc this surgery is basically the only way I will ever be NED. My tumor has taken over the vascular system in my liver.

Hubs and I did some talking, and crying, we need some more information, we see the surgeon on the 20th for the follow up. What we heard today were the results from the tumor board. Hubs has said he does not want to watch me waste away. We are leaning toward taking the risk and doing the surgery. So much to think about.

What I do not know is how involved a "standard" liver resection is. My onc stated the surgery they are planning for me is rare, my surgeon has never actually performed it but an associate of hers has and would be part of my surgery team. I am just trying to get a grasp on what a liver resection entails normally. Any input is appreciated. Thanks in advance.

⸜⸝

In spite of facing this difficulty, Beans continues to welcome and offer support to new users, as well as keeping all of us in her prayers...

Well it was an informative appointment. I did find out there would be three surgeons, one of which is a liver transplant surgeon. Should we decide to proceed I will meet the additional surgeons.

The plan for now is to complete 3 more cycles of chemo (each cycle being a set of two infusions) and have another scan to see if the tumor has shrunk any more. If it has I would do two more cycles while they get the surgery set up to hopefully get more shrinkage.

It is not set in stone yet, I still have to say yes but I am doing the chemo anyway. If the tumors shrink they may not have to do such an involved surgery. There will be a lot of thinking and praying going on for quite some time here.

Thank you everyone for all the advice and support you have given so far.

Got a call this evening from my onc's nurse. They are delaying my treatment until next week because of issues with this stupid vectibix rash. It has spread again and I have some pretty painful areas even with taking the doxycycline daily to minimize it. Now if the pharmacy would just hurry up and fill the lidocaine cream prescription I will be a happy camper.

Don't quite know how I feel about it. On one hand I am glad because this last one took a lot out of me and I had a longer than normal recovery. I know my body could use the break.

On the other hand I'm a little peeved because this delays everything else and I want nothing more than to get to surgery.

There really is nothing I can do about it. My onc has made the call to cancel it. I know I should take advantage of feeling semi well for an extra week and enjoy it.

I hate the thought of the delay, I know it is only a week in the grand scheme of things. I'm afraid this will keep happening and it will be the surgery that never materializes all over again. I know that is not fair of me to think, my doctors here are vastly different than the ones I had in Texas. I suppose I am being irrational and impatient.

Why does everything have to be so dang complicated????

UPDATES Oct 2016

Found out the oddest thing today when I went for my infusion.

Apparently my tumor pathology was redone by the pathologists when they received my tumor tissue.

They found I do in fact have a RAS mutation. It is not KRAS, my oncologist didn't say which exact one it was, just that it was a rare mutation that possibly was not tested for by my docs in our previous locale.

As a result the vectibix will not work. Kind of a bummer since the research I did on vectibix said it worked really well. I would have endured the rash for the tumor shrinking results.

My onc is also going to clarify the number of treatments my surgeon wants, he thinks they want too many and the surgery needs to be done sooner. So hopefully we will find out more after our next treatment. He is going to do the scan after the next round and we will see if we have any shrink of the large liver tumor.

Fingers crossed we get some good shrinkage!

━━ ❧ ━━

So I couldn't have my infusion today because my counts are too low. My new onc doesn't like to use neulasta to boost counts so I don't get an infusion until they come back up. He will use it if it takes too long for them to come back up but he would rather not.

Anyone know of more natural ways to boost your counts? Are there any supplements that will help?

We are going to test again next week to see if I can get my infusion. They are going to perform my surgery sooner than originally thought, I need to have this next infusion then I go for an MRI, then I get sent to the surgeon to plan the surgery so I really don't want this to be held off for too long. Any info would be appreciated.

So my counts were even lower yesterday than they were before so of course treatment has been pushed off for another week. They gave me a shot of neupogen in the office and I will be starting to give myself the 4 injections after the next round.

My onc decided on neupogen - I was on neulasta prior to seeing this oncologist. I know how the neulasta made me feel, I am trying to find out if the neupogen will make me feel the same way.

I took a Claritin but I am still having bone pain, is there something else that works with neupogen?

Any info you can provide is greatly appreciated!

I did not take the Claritin before the shot this time because I did not know I was going to get the shot. I do have Claritin D but it is the generic since that is much cheaper. I don't know if that makes a difference or not.

I will definitely take it before the next round and see if that works better. Right now I am dealing with the headache and extremely sharp pain down through my spine and in my ribcage.

My WBC's were 1.9 10*3/UL this time. The biggest problem has been my neutrophils, they were 0.60 last time I had to hold off, they came up to 1.93 the week after and they gave me chemo, this week they were 0.44 so I agreed to the neupogen. I can't keep having the delays and it seems my system just can't bounce back fast enough.

I guess I can be thankful that this delay will make Thanksgiving an off week instead of a chemo week like it was before.

Thanks for the info! Keeping you in my prayers.

UPDATES Nov 2016

Well, surgery is on hold. Tumor grew with folfiri and they won't do the surgery unless it is shrinking.

We are starting folfirinox plus Avastin today. We are throwing everything but the kitchen sink at it hoping for shrink.

It's upsetting, I was hoping to hear it shrunk and I was going to get the surgery. Now that damn expiration date is in the back of my mind. This new cocktail better work!

I'm hanging in there. My first treatment with Folfirinox and Avastin was very difficult. It made me really sick. I'm finally feeling more like myself and I go for my next treatment tomorrow.

We will have to have a frank discussion with my oncologist, either we need to manage the side effects better or we need to reduce my doses. The biggest issue is hydration to flush the chemo out of my system. The metallic taste is so bad I just don't want to eat or drink. It may come down to trying to see if I can get an infusion nurse that comes to my house to give me iv hydration. Hubs would bring me to the oncs office to get it but it would take so much out of his workday it would make things difficult.

I'm hoping everything I am going through is worth it. Hubs said seeing me so sick is very hard on him. I'm glad he finally opened up to me about it and I understand where he is coming from. I know it is hard on the girls too.

We are banding together to get through this, I just hope we can make the upcoming rounds easier.

After all of this, we were not surprised to find out that our dear Beans was feeling a little down. She, however, was surprised to feel this way. This is part of the warrior nature that is just a part of who she is. We love her, and

177

were quick to remind her that even warriors sometimes feel defeated and need a quiet place to rest.

Since I have been on here, been kind of down, reading the NED stories haven't been helping like they usually do.

The "everything but the kitchen sink" chemo has been hard on me, not as bad at the first time but still not easy. I just want to get to surgery!

Got some good news, my insurance will pay for optivo (spelling?) but I'm not sure it is as good as the keytruda. Onc said it would keep me stable, no cure but the side effects won't be as bad.

We won't change to that until we see if this chemo works. I need shrink in the worst way and the dang tumor is not listening!

Anyway, thought I would pop in and say hi, I'm still kicking, and sending prayers out to everyone.

Things didn't ease up much for BeansMama from there, but in spite of that she continues to fight, hope and pray for all of her fellow Survivors.

Wed Jan 04, 2017 -- Bad News Yesterday

Well, I typed this once and it seems to have disappeared. Let's try it again.

I have now officially failed every chemo there is. They did a CT scan on me in the hospital. My oncologist decided to use that one instead of sending me for another one next week. My tumor is so aggressive it grew on the folfirinox + Avastin cocktail. It is kind of surreal sitting here realizing that in the long run none of the chemo worked. I'm really still trying to wrap my head around it.

I am now receiving immunotherapy, my insurance company has approved 13 cycles (26 treatments) with Opdivo. From what I understood it works for 60% of CRC patients. I'm hoping I am part of that 60%. There is still a glimmer of hope left after all of the bad news. I of course will be checking those odds (me who usually says screw the odds they are just a number!) and add whatever I can to increase those odds. First addition is frankenscence oil.

Started making a bucket list and the lists of things we need to take care of (should have taken care of long before now). Going to start writing letters to the girls for their important occasions just in case. I figure if I am part of the 60 - bonus its already done!

My gut feeling isn't good, I learned long ago my gut is usually right. Not going to stop fighting though. At the very least I pray I stay stable until there is a cure. I will fight until there are no options left.

MSK logistically just won't work for us. We cannot afford to maintain 2 households yet again. Also it would be me going by myself and with my husband's work demands we would need to hire in home help for both homes as he would have the kids and I need physical help quite a bit. We don't have anyone who could commit that much time.

I am at one of the top cancer centers in Charlotte. They also refer to Duke if they feel Duke has a better treatment. I believe the HAI may be available where I am but I am not sure. I need to talk to my liver surgeon about that. She has a number of liver targeted treatments in mind last we spoke, I need to make another appointment with her to find out options.

My oncologist said that a fellow team there is starting a new clinical trial he may try and get me into. The only thing that may exclude me are the sheer number of treatments I have had.

The other issue is size and placement of my tumor. It's not your standard liver met. It is between the lobes of my liver and over 10 cm x 8 cm. Can't remember the exact measurements. The biggest issue is that all of my hepatic veins and my hepatic artery are inside the tumor. They actually just told us that it is beginning to crush my bile duct. It's not time for a stent yet as my numbers are still good but it could be needed in the future.

I wish it was in one side or the other instead of both and easily removed.

Thank you so much for the prayers. I am trying very hard to continue believing I am in that 60%. I will continue to talk with God about hopefully being in that 60%.

I am sincerely trying to maintain a positive attitude, it gets difficult when you continually get knocked down. But such is the nature of this disease and that is what I need to keep reminding myself.

I still have that glimmer of hope that the immunotherapy is going to be that magic bullet! Those prayers and hugs help me daily. I start getting down and I come here and read one of the posts or a pm you guys have sent me and it helps lift me up again.

Keeping you and your family in my prayers.

As a fellow Mom, I understand the desire to keep fighting no matter what, and how sometimes you just need to put the sword down for a rest. These words by Beans showcase the fact that this fighting nature and dauntless spirit are such a part of who she is -- are part of who so many of our fellow survivors are. We love her for it, and we're sure her family does too.

I never understand what is so spectacular about what I am doing. I would think that anyone in my position would do the same. They would fight with everything they have to try and beat this.

Maybe I am just looking at it from a different perspective, I see the weaknesses that I tend to hide from others. Maybe once I am through this everything will become clear and I will understand.

> --BeansMama
> Diagnosed at age 40
> Tumor found 9/2015

Surgery 1 - 11/2015 LAR and colostomy
Surgery 2 - 11/2015 wound vac
Surgery 3 - 12/2015 revise resection, move colostomy
Mets to liver - tumors inoperable - one tumor gone with chemo! One more to go (too bad it's the big one)
Stage IVa (T3 N2a M1a)
Primary tumor 9 cm x 7.5 cm x 2 cm
Beginning Folfox 1/2016 - Folfox no longer shrinking tumors
Lynch positive 3/2016
Beginning Folfiri and vectibix 8/2016 — Failed
Beginning Folfirinox + Avastin 11/2016

———

That is definitely my prayer for you, my friend – that through this everything will become clear, along with you getting that cure. May 2017 be a gentler year on us all.

Thank Yous

There are a ton of people to thank.

First and foremost, my most precious Heavenly Father. Without you, I would not be strong enough to either endure this journey or find the courage to write about it. I am so blessed in my life that sometimes it overwhelms me.

To my amazing husband, my super-hero and my rock, my place to land and lay down my sword and shield, my blessing from God, and without a doubt the best part of me: You teach me how to be a better me, but you never judge me when I fail. Words are not nearly enough to express how very much I love you.

To my son, my joy, my heart, the very breath inside me: I hope that no matter what else I do in life, the one thing I teach you is to have faith in your maker. Without faith and hope, we are nothing. The single greatest truth that keeps me going in this battle is that I can show you by my example what it means to know God. If I can do that, I have succeeded as your mother. I love you more than anything else in the universe. More than all the whales, and all the dolphins, and all the lions, and all the tigers, and all the giraffes and all the EVERYTHINGS in the whole! wide! world!

To the people on Colon Talk: you are my heroes. Each and every one of you. You gave me my power back when I was powerless. You share hope and inspiration along with information every single day. You face crazy odds with grace, dignity and brutal honesty. I admire you, and pray for the day when we can finally end this wretched disease. For every mom, dad, sister, brother, son and daughter who has been lost, your light goes on and brightens the way for those who follow. My heart will always be with you all, as will my prayers.

To cptmac, Lee, Miss Molly, and the incomparable BeansMama: a special thank you for being willing to share your stories with me and with the readers who will hopefully find this book. Hope is something you can't teach, and you can't buy, yet it's something you give to others every day. May God bless and keep you, my friends.

And finally, to those of you who are reading this book: thank you for sharing this journey with me. If you are reading it because you or someone in your life has been touched by cancer, I hope that it provides you with some insight, good information, and mostly hope that this does not have to be the end. As my friend cptmac so eloquently said, as long as you're alive, there is hope.

In love and faith,

Tracy

Tracy was born and raised in Central New York, where the seasons of the year are Winter, Even Worse Winter, Summer and Construction. She stays warm by writing stories, music and even musicals, but will tell you that her greatest creation, her best story will always be her family: her son, and the amazing husband God blessed her with.

Visit Tracy's website at www.tebradford.com.

Print Edition

Made in United States
North Haven, CT
19 August 2024

56276269R00114